Beauty in the Broken Places

Beauty in the Broken Places

A Memoir of Love, Faith, and Resilience

ALLISON PATAKI

Random House
New York

Beauty in the Broken Places is a work of nonfiction. Some names and identifying details have been changed.

Published in the United States by Random House, an imprint and division of Penguin Random House LLC, New York.

RANDOM HOUSE and the HOUSE colophon are registered trademarks of Penguin Random House LLC.

LIBRARY OF CONGRESS CATALOGING-IN-PUBLICATION DATA

Names: Pataki, Allison, author.
Title: Beauty in the broken places : a memoir of love, faith, and resilience / by Allison Pataki, foreword by Lee Woodruff.
Description: New York : Random House, [2018]
Identifiers: LCCN 2017058576 | ISBN 9780399591655 (hardback) | ISBN 9780399591662 (ebook)
Subjects: LCSH: Pataki, Allison. | Cerebrovascular disease—Patients—Biography. | Cerebral ischemia. | Young adults—Diseases—Biography. | Cerebrovascular disease—Patients—Family relationships. | Husband and wife—Biography. | Caregivers—Biography. | BISAC: BIOGRAPHY & AUTOBIOGRAPHY / Medical. | BIOGRAPHY & AUTOBIOGRAPHY / Personal Memoirs. | MEDICAL / Caregiving.
Classification: LCC RC388.5 .P35 2018 | DDC 616.8/10092 [B]—dc23
LC record available at https://lccn.loc.gov/2017058576

Printed in the United States of America on acid-free paper

randomhousebooks.com

2 4 6 8 9 7 5 3 1

First Edition

Book design by Virginia Norey

For Louisa & Nelson,
our lantern bearers on this journey

And for Lilly,
the light that pulled us forward

We shall not cease from exploration
And the end of all our exploring
Will be to arrive where we started
And know the place for the first time.
—*T. S. ELIOT*

The world breaks everyone and afterward many
are strong at the broken places.
—*ERNEST HEMINGWAY*

Foreword

LEE WOODRUFF

For better or worse.

SUCH A SIMPLE PHRASE THAT MOST OF US DON'T TRULY CON-template as we stand at the altar, giddy with love and surrounded by family and friends. Why would we ever choose to play out the worst-case scenario in our heads?

As Allison Pataki and her husband, David Levy, buckled their seatbelts on a flight to Hawaii, excited for their "babymoon," the last thing they could have imagined was that in a few short hours their plane would make an emergency landing in Fargo, North Dakota. Dave, an outgoing, athletic thirty-year-old, would suffer a rare and near-fatal stroke.

The Levys would never make it to their destination. Life had just dealt them a cruel and unexpected blow. Instead of celebrating the last vestiges of coupledom before parenthood rearranged their world, Allison would be sitting in a hospital room, five months pregnant, holding one of her husband's cold, empty shoes while he fought to survive.

A friend once remarked that life's complications do not end at the altar, but for many of us, it is where they begin. While that may sound somewhat macabre, from my older road-tested perch, it speaks to all of the things we cannot know as we stand, wide-eyed and innocent, pledging to entwine our life with another's. In those moments we feel the unbridled anticipation of possibility, the choices to be made, the thrill of life's blank page, waiting to be colored in together.

But there are other surprises in store, both sorrowful and beautiful. Life never moves in a straight line, constantly reminding us that we don't get to write the script. Therein lies its beauty, even in the moments when we feel uncertain, afraid, and broken.

I'm twenty-plus years older than Allison, and we first met as I exited a restroom stall at ABC News (true story). I felt an instant connection. She has a personality that you want to bottle for a gray day: crackling with energy, naturally upbeat and bright, intelligent, and empathetic. As our friendship grew, we discovered many connection points, from her younger years in Albany (I'm an Albany girl too), to our summers spent in the Adirondacks (she had visited our tiny lakeside community). We were both writers and she'd worked at ABC News, where my husband, Bob Woodruff, is a reporter.

After that initial meeting, Allison left the news business and published her first novel. We became email friends, occasionally chatted on the phone, complained when the writing wasn't coming (I complained, she kept writing). I have the most wonderful picture of Allison, Bob, and me at her book launch for *The Accidental Empress.* She is resplendent in a gorgeous dress, and, unbeknownst to us at the time, newly pregnant.

I proudly thought of Alli and Dave as younger versions of me and Bob; devoted to each other, adventuresome and supportive of one another's careers. They were in it for the long haul. Alli and I shared a love of words and writing, and yet we were social animals too, we got oxygen from spending time with friends. Each of us had always been fiercely independent, which worked well with the demanding and often unexpected hours of our husbands' chosen careers. Also, like we had been, they were determined to have a family. I was thrilled to hear about Alli's pregnancy, excited to watch such a couple experience one of life's truest gifts.

So it was with shock and disbelief that I opened an email from Allison explaining that Dave had had a stroke and they were at a rehabilitation hospital in Chicago. It was devastating to think about anyone I knew setting out on this horrible journey. This was not a curse I would wish on my enemy, let alone a young couple on the cusp of becoming parents. It seemed so unfair, both of us twinned in this horrible fate, husbands cut down in their prime— Dave, before he had finished his medical residency; Bob, before he could truly enjoy the privileged anchor chair. Meeting that day by the sink years earlier—when I was just transitioning out of my caregiving role after my life was upended by Bob's injury—neither Allison nor I could have predicted that she would join my club. The one I refer to as "the Club of the Bad Thing"—a club in which no one wants to be a member. I ached for them both.

Knowing too much about this injury, I worried how Dave would recover and what life would look like for them. Would their child ever know her father? When our own tragedy struck, Bob and I had eighteen years of marriage under our belt, four children, and a strong foundation that had already weathered disappointment and loss. I could not stop thinking about the next stage of their journey. I knew the statistics—my husband was that rare miracle in the world of TBI (traumatic brain injury) recovery. Even with such amazing progress and success, our own relationship had been strained at the seams, rearranged at times, and frayed by the roller-coaster ride of recovery that Alli describes so well.

TBI is one of the very worst tragedies that can befall a loved one. Yes, of course, there is death and cancer, dementia and ALS, an entire roster of other horrible clubs that loved ones inadvertently join. It's the "in an instant" nature of a brain injury, the alacrity with which it permanently changes and upends lives, relationships, and marriages, that is so stunning. The immediate line between "before" and "after" creates a sense of emotional whiplash. Like Allison, I was reeling for weeks and months simply trying to process the fact that my husband had been hit by a roadside bomb. I knew the risks of being married to a war correspondent, but there is an ocean's distance between possibility and reality. In 2003 when Bob was embedded with the Marines during the Iraq invasion, and for the entire decade he reported from war zones, I had contemplated death but never disability. Not at his age, not in the prime of our lives. Silly me.

Three years later, as unopened bottles of champagne sat on the dining-room table, sent by friends and colleagues to celebrate Bob's ABC *World News Tonight* co-anchor appointment, my husband lay in a medically induced coma, toggling between life and death. One morning he had kissed me goodbye, for what was meant to be a short trip to the Middle East. Days later I was being told he might not make it out of surgery, even as plans were underway to airlift him home from Baghdad. Like Allison, I would struggle to comprehend the fact that our world had been so swiftly and completely shattered.

Why is TBI so devastating? When the injured person is your husband, there is a special element of heartbreak, an unusual tangle of emotions, sorrow, and gratitude—and so much damned uncertainty. There are no percentages to shoot for, no norms, no one can tell you exactly how much your loved one will recover or how much of "him" will return. In that first year, lying beside my sleeping husband, I understood that it was possible to feel completely alone right next to the person you loved most. He was there, but not there; physically present, but with pieces missing.

It was as if he were an engine and someone had reached inside and fiddled with the wiring.

Gone was "what had made Dave *Dave*," Allison writes so compellingly in these pages. The loved one grieves for the intangibles, the inchoate part of coupledom that is as hard to define as a "great sense of humor with a good ear for music," or "that silly thing in the movie that you saw that weekend when you were first dating." Those shared experiences are what sticks a couple together, the gooey center between two halves of the Oreo.

But above all there is grief, so much complicated, guilty, unarticulated grief over being thrust in this new, unwanted direction. And because your husband is alive, because he survived, you do not have permission for this most simple of human behaviors: the space to mourn the loss of your dreams and to honor the brokenness inside. You cannot speak of this; it would be too selfish. You got him back, isn't that enough? Aren't you lucky? That ripping, tearing sensation that only you can feel? That crack inside your rib cage? That is the sound of your heart breaking.

This may seem hard to comprehend, but there were times when I wondered if it might have been better if Bob had died on the battlefield. Grieving a dead husband would take you to the very lowest place, and then you had no choice but to get back up and take a step forward. What if Bob never recovered, I wondered? What if he remained in a childlike state? What happened to love if your marriage was stalled in a middle gear, unable to move forward, incapable of going back? Those thoughts terrified me as I fought to stay hopeful, to try to live in the moment.

Beauty in the Broken Places articulates so many of the things that I—and countless others—have experienced during our unexpected journeys. Allison describes the small, ordinary moments that break your heart in the aftermath of life's challenges. I could relate to her looking out the hospital window at the clear blue sky and being amazed that the world continued to turn. I remember being jealous of all the clueless people just going about their lives, running errands and headed to work, attending their children's soccer games, buying groceries. Oh, the things we took for granted!

Then there are the painful reminders of "before" and "after." For me, it was the navy sweater I kept in the kitchen to ward off a chill. The first time I entered my house after Bob's injury, I spied it, casually draped over a chair where I'd left it during the "before" part of our lives. I burst into tears and threw it in a closet. For Allison, it was the suitcase she could not bring herself to unpack, still brimming with summer clothes for their Hawaiian vacation, or the sound of Dave's voice on the cellphone.

Like Allison, I was unaware of the trite phrases I myself had used with others in the midst of a crisis: "You're so strong," "God doesn't give you more than you can handle," and (my personal favorite) "Things happen for a reason." These "thoughts and prayers," as I began to call them, can feel like a thousand little paper cuts. I truly believe there is no wrong expression of sympathy, but some remarks can feel like pity. I liked it when people empathized, when they told me how much this "stunk" or that it was "unfair." For some, you can sense that they almost believe your bad fortune is "catching." There is a collective relief, a palpable sense of gratitude, that fate has passed over their household and visited someone else. It's sometimes hard in these moments not to feel like a circus freak, to stay focused on the positive and leave the door open for hope and maybe even a little miracle.

You discover many things about yourself in these situations, but you also learn much about your friends. Sometimes the people who show up are not necessarily the ones you expected. Tragedy holds up a mirror that reflects back all the things that can befall others. It's a special person who can show up and repeatedly walk through that door to mentally meet you in the room you are in.

And while Allison gives me a bit too much credit on these

pages, I was honored to be her "voice of experience," to offer a perspective from a few years down the road, assuring her that she would not only survive, but ultimately thrive. The truth is: it is their own grit, temerity, and perseverance that shine through in this memoir. That is what eventually saved her and Dave. Their story is a reminder that human beings are built to survive, even if the day to day doesn't look too pretty.

It was Alli's need to make sense of the world around her as a writer that became part of her salvation, and the gift she gives us with this book. I had acted on that same instinct in the hospital, almost ten years before. In a world that had suddenly flipped upside down, writing was the only way I could create order. I needed to write to help me remember the life Bob and I had made, to transcribe the events for our family in case he didn't survive. I also wrote because its very act gave me hope and reminded me of the many reasons my husband had to live and how many people loved us.

And as her own husband lay comatose in the hospital, Allison wrote: "Dear Dave . . . I love you . . . I miss you . . . May we always remember how lucky we are." My breath caught in my throat when I first read those words. Her ability to focus on the blessings and the love they shared sowed the first seeds of her resilience. And Dave's singular determination to tackle the day-to-day hard work of recovery braided them back together as a couple—and a family.

I also admire the way Allison speaks openly and honestly about faith, the places in the journey where, in the absence of anything else, the prayers and good wishes of so many people were laced together like a quilt. Faith is a powerful weapon, and in the past twelve years, visiting with service members in hospitals, children with head injuries and concussions from sports, adults recovering from car accidents, babies who were shaken by sitters, I can tell you this: people who believe in something bigger than themselves simply have an easier road. Faith is the trampoline that may not always bounce us up, but in its most basic form, it can stop us from sinking any lower. Faith allows us to believe in miracles. And who among us doesn't want that? Even for couples like Allison and David, who drew on reserves of love, faith, hope, and a network of devoted friends and family, the journey to come out the other side was still difficult. It is a journey they will always be on.

Let me be very clear: this is not a sad story. This is not a story about worst-case scenarios or even miracles, although there is very much a miracle at work in these pages. This is the story of a marriage. It's about the "for better or worse" part. It's about falling in love and joining your life with another, like two ends of a buckle, while allowing yourself to believe that you will grow old with someone in lockstep, that you will face the world as a unified front and have the good fortune to die in your sleep.

But here is the thing: all of us will have something, we will all face challenges. Tragedy and loss are the great unifiers, both horribly average and absolutely inevitable. They are the terrible club to which we will all eventually belong. We may not want to think about it, but part of life means facing struggles, confronting disappointments, and eventually losing people we love.

In the end, the details of the bad thing do not matter. What's important is how you choose to respond. It's about not letting the bad thing define you. And if we can love and hug and hope and pray and keen and write our way through the hard parts, the way Allison and David have done, then we will have triumphed in every way.

And that is the story you now hold in your hands, a wonderfully well-written, real, sometimes messy, honest, inspiring, scary, happy, personal playbook for dealing with life's vicissitudes. Al-

lison's story both teaches and reminds us that love, hope, friendship, family, faith, gratitude, and even a good sense of humor are
essential tools for recovery.

As you read this book, you will want to walk into the rooms of
your sleeping children and listen to them breathe. You may just
turn and kiss your spouse or remind someone out of the blue that
you love him or her. Hug a friend just a little longer, go for a walk
with a girlfriend, schedule that golf game, read a second story to
your grandchild. It's that kind of book, one that reminds us to
slow down, to take stock of our good fortune and the small, every-
day blessings we mostly take for granted as we rush through each
day. Yes, there is beauty everywhere. And, yes, it dwells even in
the broken places.

Beauty in the Broken Places

I BEGAN WRITING MY HUSBAND A SERIES OF LETTERS WHEN IT became clear that he could no longer make new memories. Or remember the old ones, for that matter—the ones we had made together. When Dave woke up from a near fatal stroke, age thirty, beautiful, seemingly strong and outwardly intact, he could not carry memories from hour to hour, much less from one day to the next. As his eyes blinked open, those green eyes that had first pulled me in, he stared at me with this terrifying and alien expression: utter blankness. Those were not *Dave's* eyes—those were not the eyes I knew, the conduit into the mind I knew, the mind stocked with deep feelings and well-worn love and fast-paced thoughts and so many memories, so many hopes in the present and plans for the future. No, those were just two vacant eyeballs that gave utterance to nothing more than a harrowing void, a mind wiped clean. The mind of my husband, wiped clean.

So I decided to write to him. I opened up my laptop and began typing, saving the Word document as "DearDave.doc" because that was how the first letter began. *Dear Dave, Tonight you turned to me on the airplane and told me that you couldn't see anything out of your right eye.* They were terrible words to write. Nevertheless, in some way I did not yet understand, I knew that I needed to write them. I would write it all down so that if Dave ever came back to me, he could read them. I would provide the memories that Dave could not make on his own, so that he could know what he went through. What we went through. And we could, hopefully, heal together.

June 9, 2015

Dear Dave,

    Tonight you turned to me on the airplane and told me that you couldn't see anything out of your right eye. Pupil dilated.

    In the taxi I had been thinking. Thinking about you, actually. About how much I loved you and how lucky I was to have you and how lucky we were to have each other and the beautiful and rich life we shared and the baby that was ours on the way.

    That was in the taxi.

    I'm still lucky to have you. But I'm sorry that it took you having a stroke for me to realize that. I sat on the plane clutching your shoe, still warm from the blood that pumps through your veins, thinking that, when this shoe goes cold, I might never touch another piece of clothing that is warm from Dave's body again.

Chapter 1

"Is there a medical professional aboard the plane?"

I think all young doctors live with a certain amount of trepidation about hearing this question. What a terrible summons to get at 35,000 feet in the air, removed from all medical equipment or access to healthcare facilities or colleagues to consult. The question is equal parts known and unknown: you know why you are being called, and yet you have no idea to what. What if you are a throat specialist being called to deliver a premature baby, or a dermatologist being called to a life-threatening heart attack?

But on June 9, as we prepared for our flight to Seattle, Dave and I were not concerned with anything like that. It was a glorious early-summer day. June really is the best time of year in Chicago. After our long, notoriously difficult winters—the vestiges of which can remain parked like a gloomy, uninvited guest through May—the city and all of its inhabitants come surging back to life.

It was the ideal sort of summer day: clear, sun-drenched, a balmy temperature that lures you outdoors and insists on putting you in a good mood. And Dave and I were certainly both in good moods as we hopped into a taxi and headed to O'Hare Airport.

I checked my phone as the driver weaved through rush-hour traffic. My parents had responded to an email we had sent with our hotel information and flight itinerary. Dave's mom had replied to a text message from Dave that had included a photo of me standing in profile, my baby bump clearly visible against the backdrop of the Chicago River. Dave and I were tracking the size of the baby on a weekly basis on an iPhone app, and Dave had sent out the photo with the message **"Five months, the size of a papaya!"** His mother texted us back: **"Cutest little papaya I have ever seen. Enjoy the trip and the much-needed rest and relaxation. You both deserve it."**

Dave smiled and clicked off his phone. We agreed. We were both exhausted and eager for some time together. I had just delivered a big round of edits on my latest novel, and felt as if both my brain and my body had limped over the finish line. Dave, a third-year resident in orthopedic surgery at Rush University, was wrapping up a grueling few months; his most recent rotation was a self-directed research block, and he was working on no fewer than twenty-four different medical papers. The pace he kept at work still struck me, after many years of his medical training, as untenable—he seldom slept more than four hours a night.

As we sat side by side in the cab, relieved to be heading someplace where we could sleep and relax and enjoy the rare opportunity to spend several days in each other's company, I glanced sideways at my husband and thought to myself how lucky I was. It was one of those out-of-body moments when you take a step back and take stock of the present moment, and as I did that, I thought: *I am so lucky.* I did not say it aloud, but I remember so distinctly that I thought it. I looked at Dave with eleven years of shared history to color my view—a college courtship, a young, largely untested relationship post-graduation in the wilds of New York City. And then came some big tests. Medical school and marriage, surgical residency and the illnesses of loved ones, moves around the country and a rescue dog, all parts of the life we had woven together, and now a new baby that would be equal parts Dave and me. I loved Dave as much as I'd first loved him in college, but the love was different now, more textured, you might even say better, made stronger by the fact that it was broken-in and tested and bolstered with years of friendship and understanding and so much shared *life*.

This is not some rosy retrospective—I remember it as clearly as I remember the taxi and the rush-hour traffic and the sunny June day. I remember exactly what I thought as I stared at him in that car ride to the airport. I thought, to be precise: *I am so lucky to have Dave.*

We were both in busy, hard-charging careers, careers that forced us to spend more time apart than we would have liked, and yet we could not help but feel like we were stepping together into an exciting new phase in our lives. After more than a decade of medical training, Dave was on the cusp of becoming a senior resident. After years of being the overworked underling, he was about to start reaping the rewards of his intense labor and sacrifice and sleep-deprivation. At thirty years old, he had spent more than a third of his life working toward this goal, pouring himself into this medical training, and the finish line was finally on the horizon.

I, too, felt like I was riding a wave of momentum in my own career; after two tough but successful book launches in two consecutive years, I was now working on my most ambitious, most exciting book yet. It had been a risk for me to leave my stable day job in news in order to pursue my passion of fiction writing. I had worked hard, and it was an unpredictable but exciting time as I tried to build my career.

And best of all—Dave and I were about to become parents. Earlier in our marriage, we had made the decision to put off starting a family for a few years because of his grueling medical training (plus, it was not exactly possible to conceive when we never saw each other). But here we were. We were finally ready. Parenthood was just around the corner—a little girl, we had found out the week before—and that was going to be the most important adventure of our lives.

"We are on time, can't wait to see you in Seattle!" Dave typed the text message to his eldest brother, Scott, as our plane prepared to take off from Chicago. En route to our "babymoon" in Hawaii, we planned to make a three-day stopover in Seattle to visit two of Dave's older brothers who lived out there. I had never been, and we had even scheduled a quick one-night getaway up the Pacific Coast to Vancouver.

I remember it all with such crystalline clarity: the rush-hour traffic moved, the airport security line was short, and we had a windfall of time to stop at Chili's for a quick dinner. While we waited for our food, I ran across the terminal to grab a couple of books from Hudson Booksellers, feeling giddy at the thought of vacation and so much free time for leisurely beach reading.

It was all so remarkably *ordinary,* the last ordinary night we would spend as the inhabitants of that life. We spoke about the fact that former Olympic athlete Bruce Jenner had recently re-emerged into the public eye as a woman named Caitlyn. We spoke about work and family and the fact that Dave's beloved Chicago Blackhawks would be playing in the Stanley Cup finals while we were in Hawaii. We looked through Dave's phone at his recent pictures of our sweet dog, a little female mutt whom we had left with friends and were already missing.

Aboard the plane, Dave hoisted our two suitcases overhead.

We took our seats toward the back of the plane. Five months pregnant, I was always up for a nap, so I promptly fell asleep after takeoff. A sleep-deprived resident, Dave usually did the same, having learned years ago while in medical school to grab sleep wherever and whenever he could. And yet that evening, for some reason, he decided not to sleep. He decided to stay awake to finish up some research work. We could not possibly have known in that moment what was going on inside his body, or the fact that his decision to stay awake just might have made the difference between life and death. I did not know any of that as the plane took off, leaving Chicago behind, and I drifted off into blissful, hormone-induced sleep.

I awoke to Dave nudging my arm. "Yeah?" I turned to him, groggy, unsure of how long I had been asleep. His laptop was open on his tray table. Through the window, the sun was just about to dip below the horizon.

Dave's voice was quiet, but with an uncharacteristic edge to it—a rare, discomfiting urgency as he asked: "Does my right eye look weird?"

I felt my heart tighten in my chest. Yes, his right eye looked weird. His pupil was bizarrely dilated, so large and black that I could barely see the beautiful green of his iris. But the strangest thing was the asymmetry of it—only the right eye was dilated, the left eye appeared completely normal.

"I can't see anything out of it." Dave blinked, casting a listless glance around the plane.

I sat up straighter, any residual sleepiness entirely gone. "Open the shade; see if the bright light makes it contract."

Dave lifted the window shade, blinking out at the clear view of coming evening from 30,000 feet high. Outside, the last rays of early-summer sunlight pierced a low cloud cover. Dave turned back to me, shaking his head. "I can't see anything."

Alarmed, I threw out the most outrageous, most hyperbolic

question I could think of. I went for the worst, lobbing my darkest fear so that it could be debunked with Dave's reply of "No, that's ridiculous," and a laugh of dismissal. I asked: "Dave, are you having a *stroke*?"

"Maybe," he replied, his voice eerily quiet.

My heart dropped. Dave was not an alarmist. I tend to be the alarmist, convinced that a swollen gland is cancer or a persistent cough is surely pneumonia. But Dave never gets ruffled about that sort of thing. In fact, it would frustrate me sometimes, how hard I had to work to ruffle him when I was convinced that I had some freak medical condition (I *had* accurately self-diagnosed a hernia a few years prior, and I believed that that entitled me to at least a few years of self-righteous medical opinions). But Dave rarely went for it; I guess after you've seen enough gunshot wounds and car accidents, you learn how to not sweat the small stuff.

And yet, Dave was clearly alarmed now. And that realization— that was scary.

"I'm going to get help, be right back." I shot up out of my seat and ran to the rear of the plane, charging toward the unsuspecting Alaska Airlines flight attendant. "You need to make an announcement—we need a medical professional. My husband can't see a thing, and his right eye is weirdly dilated."

The flight attendant, a petite woman with tidy blond hair and a wide, kind face, read the alarm on my features and mirrored it back to me. "What seat are you in, honey?" I told her, and she picked up the cabin phone to make the announcement over the loudspeaker, asking for any medical professional aboard the flight to meet us at Dave's seat.

As it turned out, there was a nurse seated right behind us, and she hopped into our row and began speaking to Dave. I returned to our row in time to see her questioning him: "Close your left eye, look just with your right eye. Now, how many fingers am I holding up?"

"I can't tell," Dave answered, his voice vacant, unnaturally quiet. And then he shut his eyes. Fell asleep, without ceremony or pronouncement. Just like that, he was gone. I did not know it then, but it would be a very long time before Dave came back.

Chapter 2

New Haven, Connecticut
September 2003

IT WAS NOT EXACTLY LOVE AT FIRST SIGHT. IN FACT, IN THE beginning, I got Dave Levy all wrong.

We met for the first time in the early autumn of our freshman year. "Camp Yale" is what it is called, a manic and fabulous time right before classes begin, when everyone on the freshman quad is buzzing about, wide-eyed and name-tagged, working hard to set course schedules and learn building names. All interactions in those first few weeks unfold around valiant efforts to find commonalities, exploratory questions to sniff one another out, efforts to gauge whether initial and tenuous points of connection might potentially bloom into genuine friendship.

Oh, you're from Annapolis? My roommate is from Baltimore! Do you know her?

Oh, you're interested in ancient Greek philosophy? I loved My Big Fat Greek Wedding*!*

Oh, you're on the field hockey team? I am seriously considering intramural Ultimate Frisbee.

And so it goes.

I was out with a big group of people on a Thursday night. It was a quintessential college bar called Old Blue, attached to the lobby of a New Haven hotel, with green carpeting and a big wooden bar in the center with cheesy gold accents. We were freshmen, only eighteen at the time, and so we were not exactly permitted to walk in through the front door of this bar. Our way in came instead from sneaking down the adjacent alley, hopping a chain-link fence, and slipping through the back door of the hotel. From there, after a discreet amount of time (spent hiding in the hotel lobby bathroom), we would slide our way through the lobby and into the bar, hopefully without catching the attention of the doorman on the other side. It was not a sure thing; Thursday nights at Old Blue were notoriously risky, made all the more fun by these thrilling elements of adventure and mischief and, if successful, triumph.

That night, our attempt was successful, and my friend Marya and I slipped giddily into the bar. Very quickly, Marya became engaged in a chummy conversation with a guy I had not yet met. Marya played on the women's lacrosse team, and I quickly gathered that this guy, Dave, was on the men's lacrosse team, and that the two of them already had mutual friends and experiences in common.

As I stood there, the unathletic odd one out, I observed Dave. I noted his fit, well-built physique, his quick quips and easy laughter. His interest in a friendly chat with Marya. His apparent lack of interest in talking with me. At one point he turned to me and asked: "Where do you go to college?"

I stared at him in silence, taken aback. I went to the same college he did. The college whose campus literally enfolded the bar in which we stood. The college after which this bar, Old Blue, was named. Had he really just asked me that?

Who is this guy, I wondered? "Meathead" was the common campus vernacular that came to my mind in that moment. I took him to be a pompous frat boy. You see, Dave had the strapping good looks of a hearty Midwesterner and a loud and contagious laugh, and he was generally accompanied by a cadre of other jocular, self-assured, boisterous alpha males. I, too, was outgoing and willing to chat up strangers both male and female, eager to make friends in those early days of college. So when I tried to strike up a friendly conversation with Dave Levy at the bar and he brushed it off without much interest, I assumed it was because he thought himself too cool. It never occurred to me that a seemingly gregarious guy with as much going for him as Dave Levy had ignored me, coming off as cold and aloof, because he was, well, *shy*.

Our paths did not cross again until the following year. Sophomore fall we were both enrolled in "The History of Art and Architecture" with the beloved professor and art historian Vincent Scully. It was to be Professor Scully's final year teaching the course after a storied career of almost half a century, so enrollment in the already popular class had swelled. In a massive lecture hall filled with hundreds of students, Dave Levy and I found ourselves seated next to each other.

There was an assignment early that semester in which we had to analyze a piece of furniture, a large wooden armoire, and write an essay on it. Dave and I had several mutual friends, and so we went to the art museum at the same time on a Sunday afternoon to study the armoire. Dave stood there, his face serious as he jotted down some notes, and then he used the word "looming" to describe the wardrobe. I turned to him, head cocked to the side as I thought: *Good word.*

It sounds so silly, but that was the moment when I realized

two things. The first: Dave was smart; he was not some broad-shouldered beef-head who cared about his sports team but not his studies. The second: I had judged him unfairly. And I had pegged him completely wrong.

Dave's brain—not only his brain, his *curiosity*—took me by surprise. I am an insatiably curious person, and so are the people I love most. I find it to be one of the most irresistible character traits because it carries this promise: continued learning; constant questioning; an antidote to boredom or passivity.

And the more we got to know each other that fall, the more we talked, the more I saw that Dave possessed this curiosity, this interestedness, this drive to improve his mind. True, Dave was also fun. There was one night on campus, after a party at a New Haven bowling alley, when someone pointed out the fact that Dave bore a resemblance to the Olympic gymnast Paul Hamm. Just then, Dave began to perform a series of cartwheels across the lawn. His ad-libbed routine ended with him diving, headfirst, into a nearby hammock. When I think back to that night, I remember contagious midnight laughter. I remember a lightness around Dave, and my wanting to be near that joy.

But Dave was more than just fun. I was especially surprised when I found out that Dave was on the premed track. My two roommates were premed, and I knew how hard they worked, how heavy their course loads were. Dave shrugged and told me that physics and chemistry came naturally to him. I knew that he also enjoyed history, since we were in the art history class together. And then I found out that he was taking an advanced course on John Milton—a class that I, an *English major,* had steered clear of because I found it intimidating. This guy had depth; Dave Levy was definitely not the self-involved, beer-swilling jock I had presumed him to be.

A couple of weeks later a few of us from the art history class were studying together for the midterm. Because Professor Scully was very much of the old-school way of doing things, he taped physical prints of all of the paintings and structures to a wall in a building on campus rather than digitizing them for easy dorm-room studying. The only way to study, therefore, was to go to this building, stand before the wall, and try your best to memorize each image. It was all very collaborative and old-fashioned, and you can imagine my delight when I found Dave there night after night that week.

I tried to play it cool. I tried to focus on the sprawling display of temples and churches and statues, scribbling notes and attempting to commit an endless procession of dates to memory. But, naturally, my eyes would slide around the room, aware that Dave was somewhere nearby. Studying for this midterm had gotten very exciting, and it had nothing to do with the temples or statues.

I found Dave, on the final night of that week, standing in a group before the medieval cathedrals. Someone was stumped as to how to determine the differences between Romanesque and Gothic. Dave explained how to identify the lightness and the height that differentiated later Gothic from its predecessor, Romanesque. He rattled off a few significant dates and locations that marked turning points in the architectural trends. We all looked at him. "Whoa, that guy is smart," some fellow student muttered under his breath. *Yeah,* I thought, *I guess he is.*

A few of us gathered that Friday night after the midterm in the dorm room of our mutual friend Peter. We played cards and drank beer and celebrated the fact that the big test was behind us. Dave had a lacrosse scrimmage on Sunday, so he was on a forty-eight-hour rule of no alcohol and could not drink that night. He hung around with the rest of us for hours, laughing and joking. At the end of the night, when he asked if he could see me safely back to my dorm building across campus, I did not play it cool. I gladly accepted his escort as well as the accompanying good-night kiss.

What took me by surprise from the very beginning of our college courtship was just how much I admired and respected Dave. I had never known someone so staunch and unwavering in his commitment to excellence. I had done well in school my whole life; I knew that I was a curious and conscientious person, someone who worked hard and did well, but he made me want to kick it up a notch.

Not only did I admire Dave, but I really liked him; when I spoke to Dave, I felt that he understood what I was saying. He understood *me*. It was as if we had always been the best of friends—a feeling of being known and a feeling of comfort that comes from speaking honestly and being heard. We laughed at the same jokes, we played off each other, and we quickly developed that ease of exchange that comes from a natural and mutual understanding.

By the end of the semester, as Dave and I were each wrapping up the English papers that were due in our respective classes, it was clear to me that he was a better grammarian than I was. "Would you have time to proofread my paper?" I asked him one day toward the end of the term. He agreed, taking the care to provide thoughtful and thorough notes on how he felt I might improve my paper. When he handed it back to me I stared at my paper, his comments, and then at Dave.

"What?" he asked. "What's wrong? Are the edits terrible?"

"No," I answered. "They're really good."

"Oh," he said, sitting up. "Well, good."

"I'm supposed to be the English major here, and you are correcting *my* English paper."

"Yeah?" He shrugged.

What riotously unfair genetic contest did you win to get so good at so many things? I wanted to demand. But instead, I said: "I'm just . . . impressed. You know, sometimes when people are re-cruited because they're really good at a sport, as you are with la-crosse, then that is their priority. And schoolwork is sort of . . . I don't know . . . secondary. You manage to do all of this, and do it well."

"You know I wasn't recruited to play lacrosse, right?" he asked.

"What? No, I didn't know that."

"I *tried out* for the lacrosse team," he said.

"You're a walk-on?" I asked. "But . . . but you're a starter. As a sophomore. I figured lacrosse was your life. Or, at least, your pri-ority."

"No." He shook his head. "I almost didn't make it at all. I was terrible freshman year. Coming from the Midwest? I had no stick skills, compared to these guys who grew up in the lacrosse cul-tures of Maryland and Long Island, playing in travel leagues since they were young. I knew nothing. Coach just liked me because of how hard I worked and how fast I could run."

"Really?" I asked, my whole idea of Dave Levy shifting be-fore me.

"Really," he said. "Freshman fall, Coach had to cut a handful of people. I was surprised every time I made it through a round of cuts. Finally, we're getting to the final round of cuts, and just a few of us walk-ons are still around, vying for the last spots. One morning we have a timed run out at the fields. The run is going to be no problem." I nodded as he continued. "So the morning of the run, my roommate turns off my alarm clock without telling me, and I sleep through the run. I wake up, see the time, and panic. All my teammates have already left campus for the fields. I have no ride out to the track. I have no way to make it to the run. I am going to get cut."

"But"—I bristled at the unfairness of it all—"couldn't you ex-plain to your coach that your roommate turned off your alarm?"

Dave looked at me with an indulgent smirk. "Blame it on my roommate? You really think he'd go for that?"

"But it was the truth!"

"No excuses," Dave said. "You miss something as important as a timed run, you're out."

"What did you do?" I asked.

"I hitchhiked, begged a stranger for a ride out to the fields. When I got there, the last group of guys was getting ready to do their run around the track. I hopped the fence and fell in with the second heat of runners when Coach's back was to me. I smoked the run. Coach never would have known I almost missed the entire thing."

"Phew," I said.

"But then I decided to tell him," Dave said. "I told Coach everything. I admitted that I had been late and had missed the start of the run. I figured he would probably cut me, but I didn't want to lie to him."

"So what happened?"

"A few weeks later, I made the team. Coach told me that he really appreciated my honesty."

I let this sink in. The whole story. I felt such a sense of injustice—his roommate had turned off his alarm clock! I probably would have run straight to the coach and tried to plead and explain and talk through it. But Dave had not treated it as some sob story. He hadn't wrung his hands at the unfairness. Instead he'd just gotten himself out to the field, and he'd put his head down to work hard and overcome the setback. I admired that so much. Not to mention his integrity in how he spoke the truth to his coach, even when there was little to be gained by doing so.

It all seemed to come into a clearer focus: the bits of Dave that did not quite jibe with the stereotype of the jock—his studiousness, the way he was always just a teensy bit outside the campus lacrosse clique. So many of the things I liked so much about him. It was because Dave Levy was a geek, after all, just like the rest of us! "So, then, you *did* get in for your grades," I reasoned.

"I was actually recruited here for football," he answered. "But I decided to try out for lacrosse instead. I knew that I had more room to improve in that sport."

A part of me wondered if perhaps all of this was a bit too good to be true.

Chapter 3

DAVE WOULD NOT WAKE UP, COULD NOT BE ROUSED FROM SUDden and abrupt unconsciousness. His six-foot, two-hundred-pound frame was laid flat across a row of airplane seats, a doctor and a nurse and an EMT (all passengers traveling on our flight) huddled around him. The Alaska Airlines flight attendants had Dave hooked up to an oxygen tank while the nurse held tight to his wrist, tracking his pulse. The odd thing was that Dave's vitals remained stable; he had the look of somebody taking a nap, a person at rest and at peace as chaos unfolded around him.

I sat in the row just in front, watching it all, trying to breathe. I kept hearing concerned, confused whispers from around the cabin.

What's going on?
He just suddenly lost consciousness.
His wife's pregnant.

I put my hand to my belly, reminding myself that I needed to stay calm. And yet, Dave was lying right there, unconscious. Completely unresponsive. My big, strong, healthy husband—an athlete, a man whom I'd never seen puff a cigarette, one of the most disciplined, discriminating eaters I knew, a *doctor,* for crying out loud!—would not respond to a team of medical professionals trying to rouse him. What was happening?

As the minutes passed, they tried to get Dave to swallow some orange juice, thinking that perhaps his loss of consciousness was due to low blood sugar. As they trickled the juice down Dave's throat, he began to choke, his eyes remaining shut as his entire body convulsed and rejected the aspirated beverage.

"He's having a seizure!" one of the healthcare professionals declared as his heavy frame heaved and shuddered. I shut my eyes, my body curling in on itself. *God, why is this happening? What is going on? Dave, what is happening to you? Will you please just wake up?*

I knew that if I thought too hard about any one of these questions, my mind would begin to spin out of control, hurling me headlong toward all sorts of dark and terrifying places. Places from which I might not be able to pull myself back. So I just tried to focus on breathing. *Inhale, exhale. Let the medical professionals do their jobs. Stay calm. I'll be here for Dave when he wakes up.*

At one point, the EMT tried manual resuscitation, pumping his chest with two hands, but it did not jolt Dave back to consciousness. Half an hour later, when Dave still could not be woken, we decided that we needed to make an emergency landing. A flight attendant used MedLink, an in-cabin service for communicating with the ground in cases of emergency, to find the nearest airport and make sure an ambulance would be waiting on the runway with a team of medical professionals to board the plane and get Dave to a hospital.

"Where are we? Where is there to land?" I asked, looking out the window at a world of black. The sun had set. What was between Chicago and Seattle, I asked myself—would we go to Idaho? Montana?

"Fargo, North Dakota," the flight attendant answered.

"I don't know Fargo," I said. "Are there good medical facilities there?"

The flight attendant returned my gaze. "It's our only option."

So, Fargo it was.

They had removed one of Dave's shoes; I can't recall why, but perhaps there was a fear of swelling. As I sat there, I clutched Dave's shoe like I would hang on to a precious relic. Dave's shoe. A piece of him. How many times had I stared at this shoe and thought nothing of it, or perhaps thought only: *I wish he would put his shoes in the closet.* I noticed how the shoe felt warm, still warm from his body. Warm from the blood that his heart had pumped through his veins, and I thought back to all the cold mornings when Dave had risen from bed, the night still dark outside the window, to go into work at the hospital. All those times when I had slid over to his vacated side of the bed, the sheets a cozy tangle from where his warm body had just been. And then a question popped into my head: would I ever feel anything that had been warmed by Dave's body again? If he died, wouldn't he go cold—wasn't that what I had always gleaned from the television shows and films? Was this shoe the last time that a part of Dave would feel warm? I held it tighter. *Oh God, Oh God, Oh God, what is happening?*

We landed in Fargo—a vast swath of black with just a few scattered lights in the distance. In the foreground, the ambulance lights spun, a dizzying strobe of white and orange. The emergency medical team boarded the plane and took Dave off on a makeshift gurney of sheets, his body floppy in their arms. I followed behind, still clutching that one shoe, making sure that all four pieces of our carry-on luggage came with us. I recalled a night just a month earlier when Dave had temporarily lost his keys—how frantic he had been because of the work he stored on a USB plug on that keychain, and I told myself that the least I could do for him now was make sure that none of his valuables got left behind.

I passed row after row of tight, concerned expressions, fellow Seattle-bound passengers telling me as I passed that they would be praying for my husband and thinking of our family. I nodded, dazed, thinking: *Yes, please do. Please pray for Dave. Please pray for me, because right now I am too scared, too confused, too focused on what the hell is happening inside Dave's body to have time to pray myself. So, yes, please do that.*

These fellow passengers would go on to Seattle. They would tell whoever met them at baggage claim about their eventful flight, about their emergency detour to Fargo. I believed their earnest concern; I believed that many of them would think of us and pray for Dave. But I also knew that, within a few moments of landing, they would go on with their lives, our trauma fading into memory.

The two of us would not make it to Seattle. For us, this was a horror story very much still unfolding, and our route had changed. Our route had changed forever.

Chapter 4

New Haven
Fall 2004

A FEW MONTHS AFTER DAVE AND I STARTED DATING, AN AC-
quaintance who knew both of us raised a dark specter of doubt
with an offhand comment that was not sitting right. "You and
your siblings must always wonder if people are dating you for the
right reasons or if they are just interested in your last name."

Huh. No, I had not really thought about that. For the most part,
I considered myself a fairly good bullshit detector. I had had my
whole childhood to learn. It's generally pretty apparent, easy to
sniff out the users—they make their intentions clear with their
overemphasis of your last name or the favors they ask for.

Take my first day of high school. I remember how nervous I
was—I was insecure and unsure of what to expect, as are pretty
much all freshmen, right? As I was walking into biology class, an
attractive senior guy held the door open for me. I paused and
smiled my thanks; I was so taken aback by the unsolicited act of
kindness that this stranger, *a senior boy,* was showing me. Maybe

high school would not be as intimidating as I had feared. A moment later the guy raised his hand to his mouth and, while still holding the door, shouted to the entire hallway: "Her dad is the *governor*! I have to hold the door open for her or she'll have me thrown in jail!"

Countless eyes turned in my direction, stares of newfound interest and curiosity. Some sniggered, some whispered. I think my wince was noticeable; I'm certain my scorched cheeks were. I wanted to trade places with the canned worms that awaited me in the biology classroom, pickled in formaldehyde and fated for dissection. I was a nervous, skinny fourteen-year-old girl on my first day of freshman year, just trying to find my way from one classroom to the next and maybe make a friend or two. The last thing I wanted was to be singled out in the rush of the packed high school hallway, the target of some jocular senior's joke, marked so publicly as different. But moments like this happened all the time. So I learned, at a very young age, how to carry and gird myself as the eyes fixed on me with interest and curiosity.

I fancied that I had learned how to cut through all that and had succeeded in surrounding myself with only genuine and down-to-earth friends. One of my best friends in college later confessed that she had gone weeks in the early part of freshman year thinking my roommate was the governor's daughter. I loved that. In fact, whenever possible, I tried to go as long as I could with some new acquaintance without mentioning my last name. As a kid I had loved the anonymity of summer camp—a place where no one knew my last name and I could relish a few weeks of being just like everyone else. In fact I had lived in fear each summer of people learning my full name or asking what my father did.

But now this girl had raised this question. And she knew that I was dating Dave Levy. Did she know something about him that I did not? Was she implying something, trying to gently warn me? Dave was affable and romantic and sensitive and he got me and we laughed at the same jokes—but was it all just a really great act?

I decided to investigate. My friend Peter was, like me, an English major, and we had taken several classes together. Peter and Dave had pledged Delta Kappa Epsilon the previous year and had quickly become fast friends with their similar senses of humor and shared Chicago upbringing. Peter knew I had been seeing Dave. He was in the art history class with us. I asked Peter, point-blank, what he could tell me about Dave, and whether he thought it was a good idea that I date him.

I will never forget Peter's response. "I've never known someone who so consistently strives for excellence in every area of his life. Whether it's his academics, his athletics, his friendships, or anything else, Dave works really hard to do everything well. I have no doubt that that is how he would approach your relationship."

I came to see that this was a defining feature of Dave's; he worked hard—really hard—at everything he did. A large part of this, I soon learned, had been instilled in him as a young boy. Dave lost his hearing when he was a year old due to an ear infection. Doctors believed Dave would be deaf for life, but his parents decided to have him undergo an operation. The medical procedure worked and Dave recovered his hearing, but he had lost nearly a year—a critical portion of early childhood development—and had fallen far behind the level of his peers.

To compensate for this lost time, Dave had been enrolled in intensive special education as a young boy. He went to a public kindergarten in the morning and then in the afternoon rode another bus to a school for children with learning disabilities.

When Dave was older and his former school bus driver heard from Dave's brother that Dave would be attending Yale after his high school graduation, this bus driver believed that Dave's brother was mocking Dave. But it was the truth—the same Dave he had known as a little boy so far behind his peers had gone on to captain his sports teams, earn the title of valedictorian of his high school, and be accepted to the college of his dreams.

To overcome these odds and achieve these accolades in spite of the many factors working against him, Dave had had to work his little tail off. He'd had to harness the ability to be singularly focused, hard-charging, unrelenting—and he'd never grown out of these characteristics.

"I love . . ." Dave paused, "going out to dinner with you."

It was several months after we began dating. Dave and I spent every moment together that we could. I was in love with him; I'd started falling the moment I saw him cartwheeling across the grass at midnight. I'd fallen fast and hard, which was actually very unlike me. I suspected—I *hoped*—that perhaps Dave loved me, too, but he had not said as much.

Instead, every time we did something together, Dave would say "I love . . ." and then trail off.

> *"I love . . . watching movies with you."*
> *"I love . . . studying with you."*
> *"I love . . . talking on the phone with you."*

At first I found it adorable. After a few weeks, I was beginning to find it frustrating. *But what about me?* I wondered. *Do you love me? Or am I alone over here?*

Finally, my patience expired, I brought it up. We were out at a bar one Saturday night with friends in early February. Dave said his usual thing: "I love being out with you."

"But what about *me*?" I asked.

Dave looked at me for a moment, taken aback. "What?"

The bar was loud. I leaned closer so he could hear me: "You

keep saying how much you love doing these things with me. But do you love *me*?"

Dave took my hand and steered me away from the crowd, toward a quieter section. We sat down next to each other in a stairwell. "Alli," he said, still holding my hand. "I love you so much that I didn't even know how to tell you. I've never been in love before; I don't know what I'm doing. I didn't know if you felt the same way. I've been saying these things, *I love... going out to dinner with you*... trying to gauge your reaction. Trying to see if you felt the same way."

I laughed—a nervous, giddy, bracing laugh.

He continued. "I didn't know how to make it special enough, to show you how much I love you. Next week is Valentine's Day—I thought maybe I could tell you then?"

I squeezed his hand. "You mean to tell me you've been sitting on a secret this good for this long, just to wait for Valentine's Day?"

"I just thought... I thought it should be some grand gesture..." he said. "I don't know, I've never done this before."

"I'd rather you not wait for Valentine's Day," I said.

"I guess now the cat's out of the bag," he said. "I love you. I never knew I could love someone the way I love you."

"I love you, too."

And so we fell. We fell hard. We were young, and we were drenched in the chemical flood of endorphins that comes from a new love and a new relationship. Dave's parents have since confessed to me that they worried about how in love we were because they were certain that our relationship could never last through the travails of college and growing up and medical school, and that that would spell disaster for Dave. "You met too early," they believed.

But they need not have worried. I had never known anyone like Dave. I had never seen so eye-to-eye with someone. He made me playlists on my clunky old iPod, and they were songs I already knew and loved mixed with songs I had not already known but quickly came to love. He shared my love for Elton John and Journey and Led Zeppelin, and he introduced me to the Eagles and Tim McGraw and Pink Floyd. "Great taste in music!" I exclaimed. Another notch in the plus column.

I hadn't expected it, but I was really excited about Dave, about seeing where things could go between us. I explained to my girlfriends that it was like living on a hill; I had enjoyed a fine view, but now I realized that it was possible to climb to an even higher foothold, where the view was even better. Previous boyfriends had been good guys and we had had good relationships, some better than others. But Dave was different—more complex, more of a challenge, a partner who truly made me want to be a better version of myself. Now that I knew that this view existed, I could not imagine going back down.

Salad days. It's an expression coined by Shakespeare. Cleopatra speaks the phrase in the play *Antony and Cleopatra,* commenting on her young love with Julius Caesar: *"My salad days, when I was green."* The rosy period of one's youth—the time when a person is green, raw, fresh. A time of innocence and exuberance and carelessness and, yes, naïveté. Naïveté made possible in large part because life has not yet been too long or too hard and the luck has not yet run out.

"You're lucky," a friend said to me that first year that Dave and I were dating. I knew it was true. I was lucky to have found Dave.

Chapter 5

AN AMBULANCE AWAITED US ON THE FARGO RUNWAY, LIGHTS and siren on. A full team of paramedics joined Dave in the back, and the driver asked me to join her up front in the passenger seat. Her face was taut with what looked like concern for Dave and compassion for me as she gripped the steering wheel. "We're just a few minutes from the hospital, and there shouldn't be any traffic," she told me, "but we'll keep the lights and siren on so we can get there as quickly as possible."

Once inside the ambulance and seated for the drive, I called Dave's parents. My mother-in-law picked up. "Hello?"

"Louisa?"

"Yeah, Alli? Why aren't you in the air?" she asked.

"We're in Fargo, North Dakota. We made an emergency landing." I could hear how unnaturally calm my voice was, quiet and toneless, even as my entire body trembled. We never know how we will respond to a crisis until one actually lands on us. I would have suspected myself to be shrill and hysterical, or at the very least crying. But there I was, my voice faint, eyes dry, my mannerisms blunted by shock and confusion. "Dave lost consciousness on the plane."

Silence on the other end of the phone line . . . a mother's mind racing to make sense of an unexpected and wholly unwelcome statement. "Is he awake now?" she asked.

"No."

She put me on speaker. "Nelson is here. What . . . what happened?"

"We don't know," I said. "His right pupil was dilated, he couldn't see out of it, and then he just passed out."

Dave's father joined the line beside his wife. Nelson Levy is a brilliant medical doctor and PhD, a neurologist who has spent the past forty years conducting medical research and developing pharmaceuticals. I was glad to have him on the phone.

"Alli? It's Andy." By the grace of God, Dave's brother Andy also happened to be at his parents' home that night. He, too, is a doctor. At the time, Andy was wrapping up his third and final year of residency at the University of Chicago before he and his wife, Erin, were to move with their two small children to Denver, where Andy would begin his three-year fellowship in cardiology. Andy and Erin had probably gone out to the Levys' home in the suburbs eager for a relaxing weekend with family. Familiar as I was with the nightly rhythms of the Levy household, I could see the scene perfectly; I could imagine them all gathered in the kitchen. They had wrapped dinner, had just gotten the kids down to sleep, and were probably about to settle in to watch a movie in the family room. *Well, sorry guys*, I thought. *All of that mundane stuff, that ordinary stuff, that lovely lovely normal nighttime stuff . . . that has just been blown up by what I have to tell you.*

But immediately I had a neurologist and a cardiologist on the line and on our team, and that was no small comfort. I shivered as I clung to my cellphone in the front seat of the ambulance, lights on and siren blaring, tearing across the quiet, starry land-scape of the Fargo night.

I didn't really know much at that point—I had no idea why Dave was unconscious or how they intended to treat him in the emergency room—so I promised that I would call back as soon as I knew more.

"Alli?" Andy kept me on the line another minute, the concern evident in his voice.

"Yeah?"

"Obviously none of us knows why Dave is unconscious right now. If this is a stroke, then every single second matters; we could be talking about the difference between Dave living or dying. When you get to the hospital, they've got to move, they've got to get him an MRI immediately. You insist on that, and you do not take no for an answer. OK?"

"OK."

"OK. Good luck. We all love you, and we're here for you." Andy is the fifth of the six Levy brothers, the brother closest in age to Dave, the baby. Andy and Dave, two years apart, grew up together—played on the same sports teams, had been the closest of friends through high school and then at college. I'd known Andy, probably one of the most soft-hearted and sensitive men I've ever met, from our days in college, too. I could hear the raw emotion in Andy's voice now as he choked back fear and anguish, as he juggled the dual demands of a brother's breaking heart with his medical mind suddenly kicking into overdrive, working hard to sift through the minimal data we had in order to search for answers. "OK. Call us back, 'K?"

"I will." We hung up.

A few short minutes later we arrived at the hospital. I noted, with no small amount of relief, that Fargo's Sanford Medical Center was about four minutes from the airport, as opposed to forty, which, in a state as large as North Dakota, would not have been a surprise.

Dave's stretcher was lifted from the ambulance and wheeled into the hospital. As I staggered behind, entering the front of the ER, stunned by the blindingly white lights, I turned to see one of the EMT team members standing beside me. Before I understood what was happening, the man pressed a wad of twenties into my hand and said, "We collect a fund for the family members . . . for moments like this."

Moments like this. I considered his words. What was this moment? What was happening?

He continued: "For a hotel, or food, or whatever you need." I looked down at his hand, and then back into his face, speechless. My mind had not even gotten there yet, to the fact that I would be here in Fargo, and I would need to make arrangements for myself somehow. Food and a hotel? *What is going on?* I thought once more. *What is happening?*

"We'll be praying for you, miss," the EMT said. This overpowering act of kindness brought me closer to the brink of tears, as I mumbled, barely audibly, "Thank you. Thank you so much. Please pray. Please do." But I had not cried yet; I could not. In that moment, I needed answers, and I needed to be ready and available to provide answers to the medical professionals who would surely be asking me questions.

A team of medical professionals in scrubs had assembled around Dave's unmoving body, stripping him of his clothing, hooking him up to an endless jumble of wires and cords and machines. I remember them tearing his shirt—a shirt we had gotten the previous October during a road trip to Dave's childhood summer camp in Mentone, Alabama. I recalled how excited the camp director had been to see Dave reappear after so many years, how he remembered Dave so vividly, recalled how Dave had been named "Honor Camper" and had won the camp's big athletic competition for his team at the end of one summer. How he had insisted Dave take a "Camp Laney" T-shirt with him when we departed. How he had told Dave to come back with his own son someday, to volunteer as the camp doctor. How, when we had driven back down from Lookout Mountain, Dave had told me that winning that end-of-camp athletic tournament had been possibly the proudest moment of his entire childhood. Now they tore his Camp Laney shirt down the middle, rending it in half to get at Dave's inanimate body, a strong, muscular, two-hundred-pound form that belied the shadow of death that was closing in around it.

Dave remained unconscious throughout all of this, his facial expression one of bizarrely sublime peace. I wondered what was going on inside that head. It was so strange, seeing him as if he had simply slipped into a deep slumber. How many times over the years had I seen him asleep? It had looked just like that. Couldn't he just wake up? In a testament to just how shocked and disoriented I was, the following completely irrational thought skidded across my mind: *OK, so we clearly aren't going to make it to Seattle, but maybe he'll wake up in time for us to make it to Hawaii. Maybe we will still be able to have that awesome trip, with our plans for the bonfire luau and the snorkeling and reading on the beach.*

The head ER doctor, a young man in green scrubs and with a close-cropped haircut, greeted me with a flurry of questions. What had happened on the plane? Was Dave a smoker? He had heard from the doctor on board (who had told the team of EMTs) that Dave had had a seizure on the plane—did he suffer seizures regularly? Had Dave ever had a seizure before? Had Dave complained of any pain recently? Any numbness?

I wanted to launch a rapid-fire volley of questions back at him: What was going on? Would Dave be OK? Would he wake up? But the guy was clearly stumped and clearly flustered. What was a young guy, a doctor, doing passing out on a plane? This was not exactly a typical situation for this ER doc, or a low-pressure one at that, what with the guy's pregnant wife sitting there. He did not know any more than I did in that moment, and I did not want to get in the way of him doing his work, so I did not ask the question that was heaviest on my heart.

Is my husband going to die?

Dave was wheeled out of the room for a series of tests while I hung back, curled up in a chair, my body trembling. I was so cold.

"Miss?" A nurse peeked her head in, found me sitting there alone. "How are you doing?"

I shrugged, the tears pooling in my eyes for the first time, even as the words evaded me. How could I answer that question? How was I doing? How was *Dave* doing?—that was what I needed to know in order to answer this nurse's question.

"Miss, you need to do your best to stay calm and take care of yourself." The nurse gestured toward my belly. "Would you like me to do a Doppler, to make sure everything is . . . well, so you can hear the baby's heartbeat? Wouldn't that make you feel better?"

To make sure everything is OK with the baby, she had wanted to say, but she had caught herself just in time. What must all of this be doing to the baby, I wondered, for perhaps the hundredth time. Surely my womb was not exactly the most pleasant and peaceful of environments at the moment. I could feel the stress and adrenaline churning through me—I could sense it in the uncontrollable shivering and the quivering of my hands. And so I did my best yoga breathing, trying to keep my body as calm as I could, trying to provide as habitable an environment as I could manage for my baby, given the hell in which we had both suddenly found ourselves.

I shut my eyes, and the silent tears streamed down my face. "No," I said, shaking my head. I could not do the Doppler right then. The sound of our baby's heartbeat made me weepy and emotional under the happiest of circumstances—in the obstetrician's office, with Dave standing beside me holding my hand. I could not handle that tsunami of emotions in the present moment. And, to be honest, a part of me was petrified. Why had this nurse suggested that I listen for the baby's heartbeat? Was there some risk that all was *not* OK with the baby? Would I lose my husband and my baby in one night? What on earth would I do? I could not handle it, not right then. I needed all my focus to be on Dave. The baby was OK; she had to be. We needed her to be.

In an effort to stay calm while Dave was out of the room, I pulled out my iPod and clicked on my music. I went for my go-to playlist for calm, relaxing music, a list of slow classic rock songs that Dave had made and labeled "Classic Rock Mellow," songs that he had introduced me to in our twelve years together—Pink Floyd, Led Zeppelin, Bob Dylan, and so on. This was Dave's favorite playlist. But as I clicked through the songs, I saw every single title with a fresh stab of excruciating pain. Not only were they Dave's favorite songs, songs imbued with memory and meaning between us, but the titles!

Helpless
Wish You Were Here
Comfortably Numb
Stairway to Heaven
Knocking on Heaven's Door

Are you freaking kidding me? I groaned, clicking off the music. I called Dave's family back to let them know that we were at the hospital and that I was awaiting information. Had they ruled out stroke? they asked. I did not know. Had they hooked Dave up to the MRI immediately? I did not know; I did not know what was happening. Nelson and Andy wanted to speak to the doctor as soon as he returned.

About an hour later the doctor was back, and he told me that the team had enough data to determine that there was no bleeding inside Dave's brain. This was great news! This meant that Dave hadn't suffered a hemorrhagic stroke. The only other type of stroke was ischemic, and that, the experts agreed, was very unlikely. Dave was young, healthy. He was not obese or a smoker or a heavy drinker. That type of stroke was so improbable for someone of Dave's profile as to be practically unheard-of. And besides, that type of stroke was so bad that, had Dave suffered one, he would possibly be dead already.

So then, it was something else. They would work hard to find out just what that was, but, phew, we had ruled out stroke! Maybe it *would* end up being something as harmless as low blood sugar.

I heard the exhales over the phone, the audible sighs of relief issuing from Nelson and Andy and Louisa when they heard this. Next, I called my parents to tell them the update. I could hear their sighs as well. "This is such a relief. I was really worried," my dad, the incorrigible optimist, confessed.

My dad had just announced a week earlier that he was running for president, so he and my mom had been busy lately, to say the least. This night they were, mercifully, at home in New York. Just a couple of weeks prior we had all gathered as a family in New Hampshire for my father's announcement. We'd stood on the podium with him, so proud that he was throwing his hat into the crowded ring. Dave had not been able to get out of surgery that day, so he had watched the coverage on television from Chicago. I had told him all about it when I got home the next day. We joked that our daughter would be allowed to watch television, but only so that she could see her grandfather on the debate stage. Sitting there, alone in that Fargo emergency room, all of that felt like another world, another lifetime.

"No bleeding in his brain," I told them. "Which means the only type of stroke it could be at this point would be ischemic, and that is very unlikely, that would have been so bad that Dave would probably not even be alive right now, so they think they can rule that out."

"Oh, that's so great to hear, Alli," my dad said. "Well, let's hope for the best, then." I hung up, promising to call back as soon as I knew more.

An hour later, the neurologist came in. He was a young guy, but he wore fatigue and concern like a tight mask on his face. He sat down with me in that blindingly bright ER, his face heavy, all of his body language seeming to indicate something grim.

He looked me in the eyes and explained that he had reviewed all of the scans. It turned out that Dave *had* had a stroke—the really bad, really unlikely one. Ischemic, not hemorrhagic. Why, he could not say. Dave had just been that unlucky. "He's had a bithalamic midbrain stroke," the doctor told me, with Nelson and Louisa and Andy listening on speakerphone. I could read so many things on this doctor's face as he explained: Sympathy as he broke the terrible news. Fatigue—it was well past the middle of the night and he had been called in from home. Stress. But mostly incredulity; he had never expected to see this rare stroke in such a young, healthy man. He did not understand why it had happened—he could not tell me where we would be going from here. He could not even tell me if Dave would be waking up.

We did not want to keep the doctor from Dave for even a second longer than was necessary, so we heard what he had to tell us and then let him get back to work.

Andy got back on the phone with me. "What are they telling you?"

"They are telling me that there is just no way to know anything at this point," I answered.

"That's exactly right," Andy said. "It could mean anything . . . it could mean anything from . . . my brother is going to wake up and be OK to . . . my brother is going to die."

I called my parents back, broke the news to them. "You guys should probably come out here . . . in case, you know, you need to say goodbye." I barely finished the sentence before the words faded, breaking into sobs.

"Of course," my dad said. "We'll get the first flight."

I hung up, alone once more in the bright hospital room. I was shivering. I could not make sense of what was happening. I pulled out my phone and sent out a group email to close friends and extended family.

> Subject: Need prayers NOW
> Please don't respond to this right now, I can't take calls or emails as I am in an ER and need to focus on Dave and the doctors, but I need your prayers. Dave's and my flight had to be diverted to Fargo, North Dakota, because Dave had a stroke. He is in ER now. We need your prayers. I will let you know more when I can. Again, please no calls or texts right now. I love you.
> Thank you.

Hemorrhagic stroke is usually the type you hear about in younger people. Young survivors often suffer loss of speech and loss of mobility. Many patients with this type of stroke begin their journey to recovery in a state of complete paralysis, without the ability to speak or process language. With long, grueling rehab and more-than-human dedication, many of these patients manage to overcome some, even many of these deficits, but it is a terrible fate for a young person to endure. We had been praying that Dave had not suffered that.

And yet, several hours later, once we had learned what had happened to Dave, my father-in-law, the neurologist, told me that he would have given anything for Dave to have suffered that type of stroke. Paralysis and loss of speech, he knew. Hemorrhagic stroke, the doctors and rehabilitation therapists would know how to address. But an ischemic midbrain stroke in a thirty-year-old? It was so improbable that there was not even medical literature available on how someone with Dave's profile survived or recovered from such a stroke. There were no case studies that anyone could look to for guidance. And so it was impossible for any of us to know what it meant, and what hope, if any, we could have for Dave.

Chapter 6

New York, New York
September 2007

I WAS MORTIFIED WHEN, ON OUR THREE-YEAR ANNIVERSARY, Dave sent a humongous flower arrangement to my work at ABC News world headquarters. The flowers came the afternoon of September 24, arriving in the main newsroom, just feet from where Charles Gibson was preparing for his nightly newscast. I was off in a side room editing a news clip that had to feed out to college campuses via our partner MTVU, and so a senior producer had to sign for the flowers and track me down to deliver them.

"How could you?" I whispered into my cellphone in the bathroom, my voice like that of an embarrassed teenager scolding a parent for not parking in a more discreet location several blocks away. "It looks so unprofessional! My boss had to sign for them!"

"Three years," Dave said, chastened by my horrified tone. "I thought a really big milestone deserved a big gesture. Full disclosure here: I ran it past my parents, to see if it was a good idea. And they thought it was."

And to us, at age twenty-two, it *was* a big milestone. We were one of the few couples who had navigated the shifting waters of college and then graduation and a move to the big city and life in the "real world," removed from the coddling womb of a college campus, and we were still going strong.

But our new life in New York City was not going to be merely a continuation of our carefree college days, and that soon became very evident. Dave was in his first year of medical school at Columbia, up in New York City's Washington Heights neighborhood, and I was living on the Lower East Side with three college friends, the four of us crammed into a three-bedroom apartment with one bathroom. Getting from my place to Dave's took nearly an hour on the subway. "You might as well be living in Connecticut; it would take just as long for us to get to each other on a commuter train," I lamented.

Fortunately, we had never had one of those symbiotic relationships in college, needing to be together at all times. I had a full life and so did Dave. We were both independent and focused on our various pursuits. This would, at times, prove to be one of the biggest challenges we faced as a couple—working to weave together our two individualistic natures—but, for the most part, it was a good thing. Neither one of us was overly dependent on the other. And for those years when our apartments were far apart and we were both working hard to gain a foothold in New York and launch our postcollege careers, that independence served us well.

I was working as a freelance production assistant at ABC News. Right at the time I graduated and returned to ABC, where I had interned in college, the writers' strike began and the economy began to wobble. This led to a hiring freeze, and the staff job I had hoped for had been scaled back to a freelance position with hourly pay and no healthcare. My salary was such that, even in our cost-saving apartment, I had only a couple hundred dollars left over after rent each month to cover every other expense, and lest I state the extremely obvious here: New York is not a particularly affordable city.

While I loved so much of the work I was doing, after eight months I needed a more reliable job and a salary that would allow me to occasionally eat more than microwaveable dinners, and I needed healthcare. I applied for a full-time position as a daytime news writer at Fox News.

I love stories. I love weaving narratives with the written word. My whole life I've been driven by a desire to learn people's stories, to get to the bottom of who they are and how they got that way. To ask questions and seek to understand what a person deems important. At age nine, when my family suddenly had a legion of state troopers around all the time—driving us, passing through our home at all hours of the day, accompanying us on family vacations—I earned the nickname "Little Miss Marple" because I was so curious to get to know them all. I was so eager to learn each of their stories. I'd get in the car, introduce myself to the state trooper (usually a middle-aged male), and immediately launch a volley of questions: Are you married? If the answer was in the negative, the follow-up was about a possible girlfriend; if the answer was in the affirmative, the follow-up was about how they'd met. Do you have children? Where do you live? Do you have photos of your kids in your wallet? If so, can I see? And so on.

These were the days before cellphones, and the troopers would communicate via radios using a series of numbers and codes. I listened intently, I eventually cracked their code, and it became not uncommon for me to take the radio receiver in hand and spout off the series of codes and numbers for the message that needed transmitting.

So, given these natural investigative inclinations of mine, cou-pled with my love of writing and my passion for history, I thought that journalism would be the logical career path. Working in that newsroom was exciting and fast-paced and I met interesting peo-ple, but, for some reason, writing news left me unfulfilled. Al-though I enjoyed much of the work I was doing, I was sort of a misfit in the industry. I did want to study the major events un-folding in our world, and the way in which individuals reacted to and shaped these events—but the panic-inducing deadlines and the rapid-fire pace of the twenty-four-hour news cycle were not for me. I'm far too much of a sponge—I soak up all of the good and the bad and the stress of my environment. I developed in-somnia that first year in the job; I found my brain reeling all night, and I was unable to turn it off, struggling to digest the flood of information, panicking over tight deadlines or pending guest bookings.

I was told, at various points during my years in the newsroom, the following things:

> *You need to be snarkier.*
> *You need to be more cynical.*
> *The goal here is to provoke outrage.*
> *Use shorter sentences.*
> *Use fewer big words.*
> *Get in and get out, keep it moving, fast.*
> *A sentence that requires a comma is already too complicated.*
> *Do you take happy pills?*

I had never been a snarky, cynical person, and I did not want to become one. I did not want to be mocked by a stressed-out, grumpy manager only because I tried my best to maintain a pleasant and friendly demeanor. I liked writing sentences that necessitated commas. I liked playing with words and language.

This emphasis on *fast, fast, fast* struck me as cursory and stressful. And I did not want to unlearn everything I had spent my entire life up to that point trying to learn as a writer.

I began to write fiction in my free time, almost as a way of winding down at the end of a chaotic shift in the newsroom—an opportunity to play with the big words and complex sentences and wide range of emotions and thoughts that were discouraged in my daily work.

Before long, I found myself completely consumed by this new hobby. Suddenly, I was rushing home from work to grab my laptop and get to writing. I would be surprised on the subway, at the grocery store, out for dinner, with a new idea for some scene or a character or a piece of dialogue, and I would run back to my apartment, worried that I might lose the idea before I could get it down on paper. It turned out that my desires to study human nature and unfurl narratives were fulfilled much more by writing fiction than by writing newscasts.

Energized and encouraged by this early part of the process, I kept going. Writing fiction became a secret pleasure, an indulgence for weeknights and weekends. It was the fun I got to have *after* work. But I did not see how I could actually make a career of it, or if I would ever be able to support myself through writing fiction. The words *keep your day job* rang sternly in my mind, and even though I was miserable in my day job, I knew that that was how I would pay the rent.

Dave was at medical school, wading through his own anxieties. No matter how hard he worked, it always seemed to him that his classmates learned faster, slept less, understood the material quicker, and were better at playing the game in negotiating hospital politics. It was one of the first times in Dave's life that things were not coming easily for him, and that rattled him. He was not the smartest—far from it—and that was an uncomfortable place for him to be. So, he did what he had always done to carry himself through times of challenge: he buckled down and he worked harder.

Dave suddenly had very little free time, and certainly no time for reading that did not involve anatomy or pathology or some other medical topic, and so I remember how touched I was when I found him reading the early, rough fiction manuscript I had sent him. He had printed it out and put it in a white binder, and I still have the mental image of him sprawled on his bed, reading my words.

Around that same time, I found a sticky note on Dave's computer. "She likes yellow gold like her grandmother. *Not* white gold. Likes the idea of three diamonds."

I had told Dave in passing—I did not even remember when—about the fact that I loved my grandmother's engagement ring. He had taken notes.

Dave's Washington Heights apartment was nothing fancy; it was a glorified dorm room filled with other medical students, but it was so far uptown that it afforded a dazzling view of the Hudson River and the George Washington Bridge. At night, as the sun went down behind the western bank of the Hudson, the bridge would come aglow, spanning the broad river and glittering at the top of the New York skyline. Life in those years was not glamorous, nor was it carefree—as it had once been—but Dave was my constant. His love was rock-solid and unwavering during those years of microwave dinners and first-job angst. He shone bright and steady, an unmoving star in a big, expensive city where no other stars were visible.

Chapter 7

I SPENT THAT FIRST NIGHT IN FARGO IN A CHAIR BY DAVE'S hospital bed, shifting my unwieldy body in a futile attempt to get comfortable. A jarring symphony of chirping hospital machines filled the room, the oxygen being pumped in and out of Dave by an endotracheal tube that snaked into his mouth. I was so cold. Even under several blankets brought to me by the kind and concerned nurses, I could not get warm. Even though outwardly I appeared calm and composed, my body was shaking and shivering, and I would come to realize later that it was because I was in shock.

The nurses came in at regular intervals throughout the night to check on Dave, who remained in a coma in critical condition, so there really was not much sleeping to be done. At seven A.M., when it became clear that Dave would not be waking or eating anything resembling breakfast, a nurse asked me if I would like to have his toast and jam. I was not hungry in the slightest, but I had not eaten anything since our dinner at the airport Chili's the night before—the Last Supper, I thought morosely—and I knew I needed to eat, so I accepted the offer. And then, realizing that I was eating for two and probably needed something more nutritious than toast with jelly, I asked for directions to the hospital cafeteria.

How strange I must have looked, trembling, clutching my tray as I made my way, zombielike, through the cafeteria, listlessly selecting a Greek yogurt and a cup of fruit, an orange juice and a coffee. At the table, my hands shaking as I poured milk into my coffee, I took stock of where we were. It had been about twelve hours since Dave had lost consciousness. I knew I was going to have to begin the miserable work of letting people know that this had happened. I would have to inform Dave's work that he had had a stroke and we were in Fargo. My mind still struggling to make sense of it all, I sent out a cryptic email to Dave's four co-residents: **"Can one of you please call me?"**

Greg, one of the co-residents, called first. All of the guys knew that Dave was supposed to be on vacation in Hawaii, and Greg clearly sensed that something was amiss.

"Greg, I'm in Fargo, North Dakota, with Dave. We didn't make it to Seattle." I took in a long inhale. "Dave had a bithalamic midbrain stroke." There, I'd said it, the first time those serious, scientific words had come out of my mouth—words I did not yet understand. The medical team had told Dave's family via speakerphone, and with my own family, given their nonmedical background, I had simply used the word "stroke." But here I was, trying it out for the first time. What did "bithalamic" even mean? And what was a midbrain stroke?

"Oh no," was Greg's immediate reply. Two words, but his tone said it all—his words came out tinged with disbelief, shock, and horror. *"Oh no" is right,* I thought.

"I'll let you know as soon as I know more. Please just tell the program, OK? And ask around if anyone in the hospital knows any experts on this type of stroke?"

I wasn't aware of it then, but with that phone call back to Rush

University, the wheels were set in motion for Dave's employers and colleagues to rally to find answers and to support him. Their answers would eventually lead us right back to where we began. But at that moment, all I knew was that I needed to force myself to swallow that Greek yogurt. And I needed to tell a few more people.

Next, I texted Dave's best friends. **"Please call me."**

Peter, the mutual friend from our college years, called first. I told him what had happened.

"I can't imagine what you must be going through," Peter said, a rare gravity in his voice, a voice that so often delivers side-splitting humor. "Please just let us know what we can do . . . absolutely anything . . . for you guys." There it was again, that same devastating mixture of disbelief, shock, and horror. I tried to wrap my head around what the news must have sounded like to others; how I would have felt to hear from a close friend that someone our age, someone so healthy and active and alive, was lying comatose in an ICU in Fargo, North Dakota, and that we had very few answers.

I knew that my parents and Dave's parents were scheduled to land in Fargo by 11:00 that morning and would be at the hospital by 11:30. As luck would have it, they had booked the same connecting flight from Minneapolis, and they would be arriving together. I went back to Dave's hospital room to resume my bedside vigil, accompanied by the machines' chirps and rhythmic hums.

My mind could not compute it all, could not connect the reality of the devastation going on inside Dave's head with the silent, placid image of his resting frame. He looked so beautiful, so at peace. Dave, for as long as I've known him, has always had great skin; his cheeks have this rosy flush. It had always ticked me off—the fact that he could roll out of bed looking great, even after four hours of sleep and chronic sun deprivation, while I would have looked like a haggard vampire in his place. Even that day in the Fargo ICU, his beautiful face appeared rosy and full of health.

I sat there, rocking myself as the baby kicked in my belly, making her presence known. I was grateful for those kicks, for the confirmation that she was still moving around in there. *Please God, please. I'm so scared. Please let him be OK. Please have him wake up. Please, God, hold Dave in Your hands.* I recalled the words of a hymn I'd sung in the youth choir so many years earlier:

> *Dear God, I am so sorrowful; is there no other way?*
> *Dear God, if it is possible, let this cup pass away.*

I looked up when a nurse entered, arriving on the new shift as morning brightened over Fargo. She had a soft, kind face. She looked at me for a moment and then I saw her features crumple. "Do you have someone coming to be with you?"

"Yes," I answered. "My parents are on their way, and so is his family."

And just like that, the nurse began to weep. This reaction, so sudden and raw, filled me with a leaden sense of dread. "Why . . . why are you crying?" I asked, taken aback. What did she know that I didn't know? I think a part of me was hoping that Dave might just wake up. That he would yawn and blink, look around, dazed by the foreign surroundings, and ask: "What happened?"

"It's just that . . . I know how hard this is going to be for you. And, you're . . ." She pointed at my belly before looking back to Dave. "Sorry, I've just gotten so much more emotional since having kids of my own. Can I give you a hug?"

I let her give me a hug, though this well-intentioned exchange was actually doing more to alarm me than give me comfort. She knew how hard this was going to be? But I myself did not yet know what was happening, what our outlook was—did she know something I didn't? Did this mean that Dave would not be waking up?

I'm not sure if it was right then, or sometime around then, that a bizarre thought popped into my head. I can only attribute it to the shock of the situation, the fact that I was struggling to process all that was going on. I thought: *I guess we aren't going to make it to Hawaii, even for the end of the week.* It was sinking in, in an odd and disjointed way. On the one hand, I had the very real fear that my husband might be dying right before my eyes. On the other hand, a part of me had still been holding out the irrational hope that Dave might simply wake up, that we might be able to resume our lives, even salvage part of our longed-for babymoon.

This nurse's hug shook me from that fog of magical thinking; we were not going to make it to Hawaii in two days, or even later in the week. We were not going to be going anywhere, anytime soon. Dave was in a coma. I did not know whether he would wake up. And most horrifying of all—if he did wake, we did not know what, or who, we would find.

Chapter 8

Dear Dave,

When does Tuesday stop and Wednesday begin? It begins with you, in a coma, on the hospital bed of the emergency room in Fargo, North Dakota. That's a sentence I never thought I'd use to describe our lives. You are wheeled, unconscious, to scan after scan, and I, left behind in the room, huddled in a fetal position, am wondering if you are dead or not. The doctors can't figure out what the hell is going on in your brain.

They tried several times to rouse Dave that morning. When the neurologist entered, I felt a sense of relief to have him nearby, to have him in charge. His face appeared tired yet fully focused; he asked me how I was doing and then he turned to Dave.

He leaned over the bed and pressed his hand firmly onto Dave's chest. "Dave, open your eyes." The doctor said it several times, his voice loud and authoritative. Dave showed no response.

We took turns that morning trying to wake Dave. They had me talk to him, hold his hand, apply pressure to his chest in the same circular motion, all to no avail. We've all heard the stories of people who wake from comas and tell their loved ones that they felt their presence, heard their words, even as their bodies lay motionless. In case that would be the story with Dave, I spoke to him all morning. I talked about our baby. I played some of his favorite music. He did not respond.

The hour neared for my parents and Dave's parents to land, and I kept my cellphone close, knowing they would call when they were approaching. At quarter past eleven, the doctor returned to the hospital room. "Let's try again." He took his place on the right side of the bed while I took Dave's left hand.

"Dave, open your eyes." He pressed his palm into Dave's chest and made circles on Dave's sternum. My focus was pulled away from the bed momentarily when my cellphone began to ring. "Dad cell" showed up on the caller ID. But before I could answer, I saw something I had not been expecting: Dave's eyes fluttered, blinking, and then, the miraculous happened. Dave opened his eyes. The three of us in there—doctor, nurse, and wife—all reacted with giddy jumping up and down.

Dave looked around before his eyes landed on me. "Hi, my love!" I exclaimed, staring into my favorite green eyes. I distinctly remember back to when Dave and I first began dating, how much I loved his eyes. He has these thick, long eyelashes (which I always hoped he'd bequeath to our daughter) that surround almond-shaped eyes, green with flecks of yellow. I have never stopped loving those eyes. And in that moment, looking into them, I burst into a tearful smile. "Hi, honey! You're awake!"

Dave looked at me, wordless, his expression vacant. He blinked his eyes, but showed absolutely nothing with them. I slid closer to the bed. "You're in Fargo, North Dakota, honey. You had an accident on the plane. But you are safe here. You're getting the best medical care possible. And I'm here with you, and your parents and Andy are here. They just called, they are going to be here any minute."

Several blinks. A blank expression. No words.

"Let's see if he can follow a command," the doctor said. "Dave, squeeze your wife's hand."

Dave blinked again, his expression still devoid of all understanding or feeling. I leaned closer, holding his gaze with mine. "Squeeze my hand, honey. Squeeze my hand if you know how much I love you."

Dear Dave,
   I asked you to squeeze my hand if you knew how much I loved you. You squeezed and squeezed and squeezed.

Chapter 9

THAT FIRST AWAKENING AND BRIEF FLURRY OF ACTIVITY EX-
hausted Dave, and he went right back to sleep, but not before his
parents and brother were able to see him with his eyes briefly
open. The air in the hospital room suddenly pulsed with a heady
mixture of euphoria and relief and hugs and high fives. Dave had
woken up! As dazed and groggy as he had been, he'd nevertheless
heard me and responded to my voice. He had obeyed a command
with a purposeful movement.

"He looks so strong," my dad said, staring at Dave's motionless
body as he drifted back into sleep. It was true, he did; from the
outside, the athlete's frame was still whole and intact—broad
chest and strong arms and healthy coloring. But he was intubated,
his inhales and exhales still being regulated by the endotracheal
tube. With the most basic of human functions beyond his brain's
capacity, Dave was being administered fluids by an intravenous
tube, his bladder being regularly emptied by a catheter into what
looked like a large Ziploc bag. He had developed pneumonia from
aspirating the orange juice they had tried to administer to him on
the plane, so a series of tubes and baggies was in place to empty

his pneumonic lungs. Needles punctured his skin in various places. He had wires attached to his chest and head. The clicks and beeps of the various monitors reminded us every second how unstable his condition was. His hair was a tangled mass from where the wires and nodes of the EKG had been attached. But in spite of this, his body looked strong.

We had a family powwow and decided to take shifts by the hospital bed. Not knowing how long our stay in Fargo would be, we booked a couple of rooms at a nearby hotel and dug in for the long haul. There was really no further planning to be done; it was very much a situation in flux. For me, a perennial planner, this was foreign and uncomfortable and added to the dread surrounding the entire situation; I hated being so utterly unaware of what was happening and what we could do about it. I hated not having a plan.

My family members were fielding the phone calls and emails and text messages that were pouring in from hundreds of friends and relatives, so that I could focus exclusively on Dave and his medical care. Though I was deliberately delegating that duty to others, I knew that a powerful surge of prayers and loving thoughts were flooding toward us all day. There were friends who arranged to have food delivered to the hospital room so that we did not have to leave Dave's side. There was a friend who spent hours on the phone with hotels, airlines, and tour companies to get our entire ill-fated babymoon trip refunded.

I spoke to two people on the phone that day. The first was my sister, Emily, who wept with me from her home in New Jersey. At more than eight months pregnant and with a toddler at home, Em was not able to fly to Fargo. "I just wish I could be there with you," she said. "This is all so fucking unfair, Alli; I'm so sorry." Em told me that her two-year-old daughter, my goddaughter, had been saying all day that she wanted to call Dave.

The second person I spoke to on the phone was a colleague of

Dave's. The Rush community had mobilized with gusto to try to help Dave in whatever way possible. I received a call from one of Dave's friends and co-residents, named Yale. He let me know that he had informed the Rush neurology department of Dave's stroke, and they all felt very strongly that we needed to get him back to Rush, where they have a world-class stroke team and one of the country's top neurology intensive care units. Yale introduced me to a doctor in the neurology department. This man, who knew of Dave in passing as a colleague, reiterated the desire of his department to treat one of their own. "Alli, we want Dave back at Rush. But . . . he's very sick. We can't move him until he is stable enough to handle the plane ride."

Hearing those words filled my stomach with a leaden heaviness. *He's very sick.* I knew it was true, but to hear it spoken aloud made it that much more of an inescapable reality.

Late that night, walking from the hospital to the hotel—Dave's nurse's direct line written on a piece of paper in my hands and her assurance given that it would be OK if I called throughout the night to check in—I looked around for the first time at the city into which we had so suddenly and unexpectedly dropped from the sky. It was a balmy evening in early summer, and the Fargo night had come alive, with people crowding the main strip, live music spilling out of restaurants and bars, a scene filled with laughter and drinks and carefree conversation. In Chicago, people welcome the return of the warm weather with a giddy determination to make merry—I imagined that this would be equally true in a city like Fargo. I passed apartments with lights on, television sets tuned to the late-night news or some reality-TV singing contest. I thought about all the people living their lives on the other sides of those windows. It was Wednesday, a weeknight. People were home from work, cleaning their dinner dishes, thinking ahead to the next day or the coming weekend. I envied them all.

That night, alone in my hotel room, I called the hospital several times to check in on Dave. "His face is calm, his brow isn't wrinkled, which tells me he's not in pain," the kind nurse told me. I then called my brother Ted and his wife in Austin, Texas, and asked them to pray with me over the phone for Dave. I sat on the floor of the hotel room next to the electrical outlet, my dead phone plugged in to the charger, and we prayed and cried. After that, I pulled myself up and crawled into bed.

Dear Dave,

I had a dream last night that you told me Jesus was holding you by the hand, and you told Jesus about the situation: you had suffered a stroke on an airplane. Your wife was expecting a baby, our first.

"Yes, I know you," this dream version of Jesus told you. "I'm familiar with your story. And let me just tell you that I've received more prayers for you than I've ever received for anyone. I hear, and I'm on the case."

I awoke feeling comforted by that dream. I had a sense of peace that Dave and I were being supported from around the world by the thoughts and prayers of so many loved ones. If ever the power of prayer could work its magic, as I believed it could, then surely we had a very strong chance of getting to the ear of God.

The next morning I found Louisa by Dave's bed, her head down on his leg, looking like she was asleep. I stepped into the room and she turned toward me. "Were you sleeping?" I asked.

"No." She shook her head. "I was just praying."

I slid a chair beside her and stared at Dave's motionless body. He was in a loose-fitting hospital gown, intermittent splotches of blood caked on his skin from all of the needles that had pierced him. I stared at those blood splotches, their color varying from a rusty brown to a startling scarlet, depending on how recent the pinprick was. As an English major in college, I had been especially drawn to Shakespeare. In Shakespeare's plays, there is so much emphasis placed on blood—not in a ghoulish, grisly, Halloween-corpse sort of way, but, rather, through the themes of family lineage and inherited grudges and the questions of legitimacy and power. King Henry V marries a French princess—the daughter of an erstwhile enemy—because she holds the blood of France's royal family in her veins and he hopes that their union might heal a war-torn England. Hamlet is at risk from his evil uncle Claudius because he carries the blood of the murdered king, his father, within. And, of course, the play *Romeo and Juliet* sees so much blood spilled over inherited grudges passed between families over multiple generations. Even a comedy like *As You Like It* sees the heroine, Rosalind, forced to flee to the Forest of Arden because she is the legitimate heir, through her blood, to her father's duchy.

And it's not just Shakespeare; everything from the Bible to *The Lord of the Rings* to *Game of Thrones* takes up these themes. Even the Harry Potter books deal with the issue of bloodlines and legitimacy and heritage and power. Hermione is not born of pure wizarding stock, so she is derided as a "Mudblood." Members of the Weasley family are labeled "blood traitors" because they, though pure of blood themselves, are willing to associate with those who are not.

I really hate having blood drawn and I pretty much hyperventilate whenever I see needles, but these themes are something I've always found interesting in literature and history. It's why Anne Boleyn was murdered—she couldn't produce a male heir to carry on her husband's bloodline. It's why wars are started and why relatives kill one another and why families and kingdoms so often rip apart. It's something that comes up in literature and history all the time.

That morning in the hospital room in Fargo, seated beside Dave's mother and staring at the stains of blood on Dave's body, I thought about this. I thought about how blood, like so much else, is passed from one generation to another. Dave had already imbued my baby with half of her genetics; that was a done deal. Regardless of what happened with Dave, if the rest of the pregnancy went smoothly, there would be a baby born four months after the stroke who would have Dave's blood pumping in her veins, and that was something in which I did take comfort. But there was *so much more* that I wanted Dave to give to our baby. I wanted her to know him and love him. I wanted him to help me raise her and love her and teach her. Dave needed to wake up, to be *Dave,* so that our daughter could have more than just the blood and genes that he had already given to her.

I turned to my mother-in-law, both of us staring at the bloodstains, and I said, "That is the same blood that my daughter will have."

Louisa nodded. Perhaps she found the comment a bit odd, as well she should have, but she did not say so.

I asked: "Can we pray together?" She nodded. We took hands and prayed aloud, taking it in turn. Afterward, I played some hymns on my iPhone and we sang to Dave.

I believe I won the parental lottery not once but twice. My mother-in-law is the kindest, strongest person I know. Born and raised in Birmingham, Alabama, Louisa is equal parts Southern belle and rock-solid steel magnolia. Louisa never does anything but the right thing—she is literally *always* thinking about the other person, sometimes to the detriment of her own interests. I've never known anyone who loves as self-sacrificially as she does.

My father-in-law is a man of science. His nickname is "Nitro Nelly" because, at the age of ten, Nelson brewed himself a batch of homemade nitroglycerine—TNT—from a child's do-it-yourself chemistry kit and proudly brought it into school for show-and-tell. Nelson is a frank and rational man of honesty and character, a black-or-white realist. My mother-in-law is a woman who sees and loves and understands everybody's shades of gray. They are a case of opposites attracting in the best way possible. The pragmatist and the optimist. Louisa is the rock of her family, and her greatest joys in life are her children and her grandchildren. I realized something right then: I was Dave's wife, I was the one for whom people were worried, but his mother was hurting just as much as I was, perhaps even more. This was her baby. This was *her* blood. I could not have asked for anyone better to be by my side and, more important, to be by Dave's side. After all, Dave had joined me in creating the life that grew within my own belly at that very moment, but thirty years earlier, Louisa had been the one to give Dave *his life and his blood.* She and Nelson were in this with me and for Dave in a way that nobody, probably not even I, could understand.

Chapter 10

BY OUR THIRD DAY IN THE ICU, THOUGH DAVE WAS STILL IN-tubated and mostly unconscious and hooked up to more wires than a computer, the medical team determined that he was stable enough to be transferred by air ambulance from Fargo to Chicago, where Dave's colleagues at Rush were chomping at the bit to treat him. Two people could fit in the plane with Dave and the EMT team, so we decided that his father and Andy would fly with him; these two would be on hand in case something went wrong medically during the flight. I would fly with Dave's mom and my parents on a commercial flight at the same time.

As we packed up the hospital room, I remembered a story Dave had told me about getting reamed out by a senior surgeon because he had not removed a patient's wedding ring in the ER. If the patient had experienced swelling while still wearing the ring, that ring would have caused loss of blood flow and eventually necessitated amputation of the finger. What if there was an emergency while Dave was on the plane? "Andy, do you think we should remove his wedding ring?"

"Probably not a bad idea," Andy agreed.

But what would we do with the ring? How would we ensure that it got safely from Fargo to Chicago? I didn't have a chain to wear it around my neck, and none of my fingers were the right size. "Would . . . would you just wear it?" I asked Andy, somewhat embarrassed to have to ask such a thing.

Andy nodded and slid it on his right hand, and we made some cheesy joke about how others might perhaps assume he was polygamous.

My father had been scheduled to be in New Hampshire that day for several campaign events. Evidently, since he was in Fargo with me, that was not happening. The press had already begun to speculate as to why he had canceled his New Hampshire events, and the rumor mill was churning at full throttle: was Pataki dropping out? Ever the sensitive and thoughtful papa bear, my dad cleared it with me before issuing a statement suspending his presidential campaign and explaining why. Within a matter of minutes, the national news outlets picked up the story and the news spread. Reactions began pouring in from an ever wider circle. One of my dad's rivals on the trail, Jeb Bush, called to let us know that he and his family were praying for us. My Twitter feed exploded. Prayers and well wishes began lighting up our cellphones. My sister had them saying mass at the Vatican, our good friend Herman Friedman had them dedicating prayer services in Jerusalem. Friends in California had an entire nunnery devoted to our cause; family members in Texas had organized a prayer chain to go around the clock.

I cannot really explain the odd tangle of feelings I carried with me in those first few days. I was so scared—scared that Dave would not be OK. Scared that whatever had caused this the first time might happen again, and that then he might not ever wake up. Scared that life as we knew it was suddenly gone. I was so sad. There were a few times when I just folded into my mother's or father's or Louisa's or Nelson's arms and wept. At one point I asked my mother if I was going to be a widow, if my baby would grow up without ever knowing her father, without knowing how excited he had been to meet her. The scene from *Gone With the Wind* flashed across my mind, an overwrought Scarlett O'Hara dressed in black, weeping to her mother, "I'm too young to be a widow."

But for much of the time I was in this odd state of calm. Maybe it was denial; maybe it was shock. Probably a sizable dose of each. But I also just had this conviction in my gut that we had so many good people on our side. We were making our case to God with as much gusto as was possible. Our prayers were being heard. And, with Nelson and Andy at the helm, we were tackling everything on the medical side as best we could. Our friends in medicine from Columbia and Rush and around the country were researching and working on Dave's behalf. I knew that Dave was enveloped in this unbelievable cocoon of love and support and advocacy and positivity. I was scared and sad and distressed, yes, but as bizarre as this may sound, I also felt confident and grateful and at peace; I believed that, somehow, Dave would get through it—that we would all get through it.

As we made our way through security at the Fargo airport, stopping at Subway to grab lunch, I remember thinking how odd it was: we never forgot for a second where we were or why we were there, and yet we were talking about normal things. We were talking about the taste difference between regular and low-calorie baked potato chips. My mom was explaining to us why she liked her brand of suitcase more than the others she had owned. A casual observer would never have known that we were flying alongside our family member who was barely clinging to life.

I looked out the window for the entire two-hour flight, my eyes searching the clouded skies for the companion plane that I knew was carrying Dave in the same direction. When we landed, I got a text message from Andy that Dave had been awake for much of their flight. Andy had explained to him where he was and what had happened and why we were heading to Rush. He had asked Dave if he understood, and Dave had nodded.

In the car from the airport to Rush, I was agitated. It was rush hour, and we were moving very slowly. "He's awake and I'm missing it! What if this is his first memory and I'm not there? I'm not there to comfort him."

"Alli," my dad said, his tone gentle, "if Dave is alert enough to be wondering where you are, believe me, that is a good thing. That's not a reason for you to be upset; that's a moment we all hope for."

We arrived at Rush and joined Dave in his room. How odd it was that our circumstances had led us back to that place where Dave had spent so much time, only now he was there not as a doctor but as a patient.

We met up with Dave's brother Mike and other members of the immediate family in a large room that the hospital had reserved for us so that we'd have a place to congregate. My niece and nephews bounced around that large family room, delighted at being all together in this new place, at the prospect of so much adult attention. Three little ones whose giggles and innocence now filled the room with an almost festive, family-reunion type of feel.

One of the toddlers was jumping on the couch while the other one darted around the furniture. I was distracted and sad and exhausted and able to focus only on the questions surrounding Dave. The congenial, baby-filled family-reunion vibe felt all wrong to me. I could not play and laugh with those little ones as I had done the previous time I had seen them, just a week earlier. I could not carry myself upright and answer people's well-meaning questions of how I was doing or make small talk as if things were all right. Things were not all right; my entire life had just been blown apart, and I had no idea how or if I would ever be able to put it back together. I excused myself and returned to Dave's empty hospital room, where I would wait for him to be rolled back in from his latest battery of tests and scans.

Standing alone in that room, looking out over the city as I awaited Dave, I remember thinking: *We're home, we're back in Chicago, now what?* This was not some temporary thing that, like the hotel room in Fargo, could eventually be checked out of. This was reality—a new, grim, entirely unwelcome reality. A reality we had not expected or wanted any part of, and yet we could not escape.

Chapter 11

New York

2009

DAVE FIRST RAISED THE TOPIC OF GETTING ENGAGED IN THE summertime, just as I was about to move out of my crowded, girlfriend-filled apartment on the Lower East Side and into a place of my own.

We were out to brunch at our favorite spot, a hole in the wall on the Lower East Side called Mud, loved by New Yorkers for its strong coffee and heaping servings of eggs. Since I was moving in by myself, I think the conversation naturally turned toward when we could see ourselves living together, taking our relationship past the realm of simply dating and into more serious, more grown-up waters. Dave floated the topic of engagement gently across the brunch table, just barely dipping his toe in the water. I remember gulping in a big breath, the alarm probably apparent on my face, as I tried to redirect the conversation.

"You realize you *are* going to have to let me talk about it at some point?" he said, his eyebrows lifted. "Getting engaged . . .

getting married." When Dave knows what he wants, he knows. Left up to him, he would have the same meal day after day for lunch—he has never wavered in his loyalty to that turkey sandwich. I am not comparing myself to a turkey sandwich; I am simply making the point that the man knows what he wants and that is that. If I were allowed only one word to describe Dave Levy, it might very well be the word "steadfast." He had never wavered in his steadfast love for me.

Dave had once referred to me, in a moment of enamored and doting infatuation (sigh, those are the days, aren't they?), as his "bride," and I had told him it freaked me out. I felt so young. I felt so immature. I felt hardly ready to be somebody's bride, let alone wife.

A huge part of my hesitation came from the fact that I felt that we both had a lot of growing up still to do. We had only been out of college a few years. Most of our peers and friends were nowhere near thinking about marriage—most were still very much single. I worried that we were so young, so immature. So unsettled in that massive city and the indeterminate period of our mid-twenties.

To complicate matters further, both Dave and I were unhappy in our day jobs, and that could not help but bleed over into our relationship. Medical school was proving to be the greatest challenge of Dave's academic life, and he was regularly stressed or exhausted, usually both. Gone were the days of carefree college life, when his biggest stress was an upcoming lacrosse game or a tough organic chemistry test. Now, a few years away from applying to medical residency programs, the stakes were as high as they could be—people's lives literally hung in the balance—and Dave felt an intense pressure to do well so as to afford himself options in the next step of his training and his career.

I continued to be unhappy in my job in news. It was not the right fit for me, and the longer I stayed, the unhappier I grew. I

knew I wanted to quit my job and write novels. I also still clung
to a dream I'd long nurtured: at some point, I wanted to live in
Paris. But could I make those things happen if I was married to
Dave? As a wife, I would have to consider someone else's interests as equally important to—perhaps sometimes even *more* important than—my own. Was I ready to do that? Was I ready to be
done with "my" turn, to shift gears from self-interest to *our* interest?

Before I was ready to think about knitting my life with someone else's, I knew that I had to get myself on firmer ground. For
starters, I had to sort out my job situation. I had worked in news
for only a few years, but it was long enough for me to determine
that journalism was not for me. After several years of writing fiction in my free time, I was more excited about that than ever. I
had two completed manuscripts, and I was speaking with several
literary agents about representation. I wanted to quit news and
give fiction writing a real shot.

I began seriously considering the idea of quitting my job and
moving to Paris. I had been invited to France for a cousin's summer wedding. My aunt Tessa told my mom about an upcoming
move she was planning for her family from Geneva to Paris—
they had an apartment in Paris that they would not be occupying
until the fall. It was available, then, for the spring and summer!
The stars seemed to be aligning too perfectly. What about leaving
my job in the spring and relocating to Paris for a few months
before the summer wedding? I had been saving for such a possible job shift, and, between Aunt Tessa's generous hosting plus my
savings and what I could earn by subletting my New York apartment, I could make it until the fall, when I would need to return
to New York and find another way to support myself.

A well-meaning girlfriend reacted to this plan over dinner one
night, asking: "Don't you worry about what would happen to
your relationship if you moved to Paris?"

It had not even occurred to me to worry about my relationship. Dave had lived in Guatemala the previous summer as part of a medical internship, and it had been difficult to be apart for months, to be sure (I remember how I would cross the days off the calendar each night, thinking that I was one day closer to having him back), but the distance had never posed any sort of existential threat to our relationship. And this separation would not, either. Dave was my roots. Dave grounded me even as I fantasized about flying far away. I would come back in the fall and Dave would be there; his love was what was allowing me to dream about these dramatic changes.

I realized then that it wasn't *in spite* of Dave that I wanted to do these things; it was *because* of Dave that I could even imagine doing these things. Because of Dave, I felt confident enough to quit my stable job and move to Paris. To try to make my vague and indeterminate career dreams a reality. To risk so much and somehow believe that it would be OK. Dave was the stability that allowed me to feel safe, even as I embraced complete upheaval.

I realized then that although I still had a lot of growing up to do, in everything worthwhile I imagined doing in my life, there wasn't a single bit of it that did not involve Dave. The thought of Dave not being there was absurd, preposterous. Like not having air. There was no version of life that I wanted to live that did not have Dave in it, right beside me.

Chapter 12

Dear Dave,

I have been so non-responsive to the thousands of people who are reaching out. Prayers flooding in. So today I wrote a long email. I sat down at eight A.M. to write one email. But then the day happened. You surprised everyone. Nine hours later, when I sat back down to write the same email, it was a completely different note than the one I had thought I'd be writing this morning.

Friday marked our first full day in Chicago in the Rush ICU. Thinking that when I got into the hospital early that morning I would find Dave asleep, I planned to write a mass email to friends and family to let them know that he had been moved from Fargo back to Chicago and we were settling in with our team of excellent doctors. I had not so much as answered an email or phone call or text message since Dave's stroke on Tuesday, and I knew that there were people around the world eager to hear how he was doing.

That morning before going into the hospital, I prayed that the day ahead would see Dave opening his eyes and displaying some acknowledgment of his loved ones. I wondered, in the taxi en route to Rush, if that might just be a way of setting myself up for disappointment. So far, he had been able to keep his eyes open for only very brief periods; he was still unconscious the vast majority of the time. No one knew when he would be really "awake," when he would begin to show recognition of his loved ones or glimmers of his former self. *Just remember,* I told myself, stepping out of the taxi, *I can hope for it, but it might not happen. Be prepared for that.*

I rode the elevator up, made my way down the hall, and turned the corner into Dave's hospital room. There, to my utter shock, I found Dave sitting upright in bed, his green eyes wide open. He looked at me intently, watched me as my face exploded into a smile. "Hello, my love!" I practically shouted.

I took his hand and gave it a squeeze. Then the nurse asked him who I was, and, to my complete amazement, Dave replied with a smile: "Alli."

"And who is Alli?" the nurse asked.

He paused briefly, then answered: "My wife."

"How long have you been married?"

"Four years."

I was elated; I had not believed that speaking would be a possibility for weeks, frankly, if ever. I had not known whether he would remember me. I had not known what to expect. So this was a moment of pure and stunning exultation.

My conception of stroke patients, the common reality for many stroke patients, is one of partial or complete paralysis. I pictured Dave unable to walk or move his hand. I pictured half of his face drooping, his words slurred and jumbled.

But this was not the type of stroke that Dave had suffered. His stroke had not produced uncontrolled bleeding in his brain; his stroke had depleted oxygen to his thalamus, and he would be most plagued by cognitive, as opposed to physical, deficits.

Physically, Dave remained strong, and we were all thrilled as we saw evidence of his strength that day. He took a few steps with a walker that morning and stood up to brush his teeth. That afternoon he made a slow but full lap around the hospital floor. He answered questions on Chicago sports trivia, identified several loved ones in photos, and even read a couple of sentences off a paper.

Because of all of this, we were busy all day and I did not end up finishing the mass email until that evening, now an email in which I was able to recap the day's triumphs. It closed with:

> All of this just reaffirms in my mind that Dave is the strongest, most hardworking, most determined person I know, and I am so amazed by him. And that the prayers you've all been sending to Dave from around the world have been working miracles in conjunction with these brilliant medical professionals.
>
> This is a marathon, not a sprint. There will be encouraging days and then there will be days that are tough and scary. Swelling for an injury such as Dave's stroke usually peaks at about day 5, and swelling is inevitable, so it is likely that we will experience some setbacks as we hit days 4, 5, 6 in the next few days. So, please please continue to pray for Dave. Send all positive thoughts his way. Keep the love coming, because we truly feel it, and we cannot wait for Dave to be alert enough to share in all of your loving prayers and words.

In spite of the upbeat tenor of that email, there was still so much uncertainty. Dave's father, being a neurologist and a self-avowed pessimist and, as he said, "someone who knows too much to know how bad it is," reminded us that these early achievements, while *encouraging,* were not necessarily *surprising.* The part of the brain damaged by Dave's stroke, the thalamus, did not regulate his motor skills, and so it made sense that Dave still had many physical capabilities and strengths.

What we should be worried about, Nelson warned, were the cognitive deficits. The thalamus can be thought of as the brain's "Grand Central Station," or the "quarterback," as it plays a part in coordinating pretty much everything the brain does. All of the data moving in Dave's brain, the "trains," could still come and go, but without their Grand Central Station, there was no place for these trains to connect.

Andy explained it to us this way: think of Dave's brain as a computer. The hard drive (the long-term memory, all of the information that had already been stored over Dave's thirty years of life) was still in there, but the computer's software that connects all of the data and allows it all to work together—the thalamus—had been wiped out. Data coming in and out did not make sense. His "hard drive" was suddenly stranded way back in his brain, unable to output all of the data that it had spent thirty years accumulating. That explained why, earlier that day, Dave had not been able to provide the word for "pen" when his doctor had asked him to name the object. But perhaps even more frightening: Dave could not hope to put in or store new data, either, without a healthy thalamus. Without his brain's "software" up and running, my husband would not be making any new memories.

Losing the thalamus was a devastating blow. One of our doctors at Rush told us: "Pretty much any medical student knows that, when asked on a test 'Which part of the brain controls x or y function?' they can answer 'Thalamus.' It will pretty much always be correct. The thalamus is basically involved in everything."

And there was something else: Dave's type of stroke, and specifically the instance of it occurring in a patient of his age and profile, was so rare that there was scant medical literature on similar cases, and there was almost no established research on what the recovery or rehabilitation should look like.

Dave had survived, but his thalamus had two huge holes in it, two harrowing graveyards of dead neurons. And those neurons were, in large part, what had made Dave *Dave.* We did not yet know what of Dave remained, what through time and rehab could be regained, and what had been lost forever.

Chapter 13

Upstate New York
2010

MY GRANDMA PEGGY IS SENSITIVE AND SWEET, BUT SHE'S NOT always subtle. And Grandma Peg most certainly was not subtle when it came to Dave, nor did she hide the fact that she loved my boyfriend.

In college, during one of Dave's trips to my parents' home, we had a nice visit with Grandma. Peggy is my father's mother, and for most of my childhood, after my grandpa passed away, she lived adjacent to my parents' home, an ever-present fixture of unconditional love and stability for all four of us children. The daughter of an Irish immigrant mother and an Italian immigrant father, Grandma Pataki grew up with so little that her life's purpose became to support and provide for the future generations of her family. Her own lifetime of hard work and self-sacrifice was worth it to her because our success was her success, our joy her joy.

During this one particular visit, Grandma was in the kitchen, cooking eggs for me and Dave (her love of frying eggs was a remnant of her years working the night shift in a diner during the Great Depression as a teenager). "Snap a picture of us," Grandma said, a coy smile turning up her ninety-year-old features as she put down the spatula and wiped her hands. "I want a picture with David."

"OK," I said, hoisting the nearby camera. Grandma then sidled up to Dave, folding into his arms. Dave returned the gesture, wrapping his arms around her, and the two of them were soon knit in an embrace entirely fitting for a prom pose or a honeymoon snapshot. Grandma had a girlish glimmer in her eyes—that was often the case when Dave was around.

They loved each other, Grandma and Dave. They did right from the start. "Your grandma is the first member of the Pataki family to truly welcome me in, to make me feel like I'm a part of the family," Dave confessed to me.

I was glad of it; in winning Grandma's glowing approval, Dave had unknowingly cleared a major hurdle. My grandma has always held a special place in my heart—a kindred spirit of sorts. A soul mate to predate the compatible soul-pairing that Dave also offered to me. So I loved that two of my kindred spirits found such an easy and natural affection in each other.

"When are you two going to get married?" my grandmother took to asking me whenever I came home and Dave was out of earshot.

I would roll my eyes, smiling exasperatedly at Grandma as I answered: "It's the twenty-first century, Grandma. People don't get married as young these days."

"Why not?" Grandma would shrug. "A man who smiles at you like that? Don't let him get away."

The years went by. We graduated from college. Dave slogged his way through the early years of medical school. "When are you two going to get married?" Grandma would ask every time she saw me.

"Not while he's in medical school," I answered.

"Why not?" she'd ask.

"Medical school is just so hard. He's working so hard. He's still a student."

So then Grandma's question became, at every subsequent visit: "How long until Dave finishes medical school?"

Subtle? Not entirely.

"Grandma, how did you know that you wanted to marry Grandpa?" I asked one afternoon.

She thought about it a moment, her eyes wandering toward the rows of old black-and-white photos, images of her as a smiling girl, a bride, a young mother, a grandmother and then a great-grandmother. "You reach a point," she said, "when you realize that you just don't want to imagine life without him."

"You felt that way?" I asked.

"Oh, sure. Besides," she said, shrugging, "I knew that he could not live without me."

Finally, on one visit, Grandma put aside even the pretense of subtlety. "How long until he's done with medical school?" she started in.

"A couple of years," I answered, knowing what she was really thinking.

Grandma's eyes went wide. "A couple of *years*? You're not going to make him wait that long, are you?"

"Why not?" I asked. "What's the rush? We're so young."

She knit her hands together, rubbing the crinkled ring finger on which she still wore the small diamond my grandfather had given to her so many decades before. "Alli, when you have a guy like Dave, you have to appreciate what you've got. Don't wait too long. Some other girl might come along who sees how great he is, and he might realize that he's tired of waiting."

It sounded quaint and archaic, precisely the type of cautionary advice one might expect from a grandmother who courted and married during the Great Depression, before women had won widespread opportunities for higher education or careers of their own. But even as I chuckled, shrugging the warning aside, I did notice a slight uptick in my pulse.

Someone else? Someone else for Dave? Dave deciding to marry someone other than me? Was such a thing possible? The thought filled me with panic. I didn't want to think of it. *You reach a point when you realize that you just don't want to imagine life without him.*

I didn't want to imagine a life in which Dave was with anyone but me, or me with anyone but him. I had always just assumed that it would be us. I had always taken it as a given, even as I'd brushed Grandma's questions and hints aside.

Maybe Grandma was more right than I had realized—maybe with her age and her wisdom she knew something I didn't. Maybe when it came to choosing a life partner, it was important not to take anything, especially the other person, for granted.

Perhaps Grandma had seen Dave and picked him for me, even before I'd known to pick him for myself. One thing I knew for sure, thanks to Grandma: I realized then that I *did* want to marry the guy. More than I had admitted to my grandmother—or to myself.

Chapter 14

I DISCOVERED VERY QUICKLY THAT THE DAVE WHO WOKE UP in the neuro-intensive care unit at Rush Hospital was not my husband. Without his mind's Grand Central Station, the "trains" in Dave's brain not only were not making it to their destinations—they appeared to have been run off the rails.

Dave was completely disoriented, medically classified as in a state of amnesia. Most of his attempts to speak were jumbles of incoherent babble. "Confabulation" was what his doctors called it. It was incredibly sad; it was also incredibly frightening.

Dave and I had always "gotten" each other; this mutual understanding had been one of the main qualities that had drawn us together. At first, it allowed us to form a quick and natural connection. Over time, this mental and emotional intimacy had produced a language of our own—a shorthand that we often fell back on without even being aware of it, comprising and woven from inside jokes and shared experiences and an intrinsic understanding of the other's mind. A close friend once observed: "You talk to each other a certain way that's different from how you talk to other people."

Well, not any longer.

Most of the time, though his hospital room was filled with close family and loved ones, Dave did not attempt to speak. When he did, I could not understand what he was saying. I had never paused to think about how much I had taken Dave's words and his mind and his very essence for granted. Not until those pieces of Dave were gone, bruised and battered in a traumatized brain, did I realize just how fundamental they were to our relationship and our life together.

It was scary to see my brilliant husband's body and mind kidnapped by this new, helpless, disoriented foreigner. One of Dave's early attempts at conversation included a long, rambling monologue in which he told those of us assembled beside his hospital bed, in barely audible language, that he had taken on all of the pain and sins of everyone else in the world, and that he had to die as a result. It sounded like a bizarre and macabre mash-up of the theology you might hear if a schizophrenic was delivering a church sermon.

"No, you don't have to die. You're wrong," Andy said, looking squarely into his younger brother's eyes.

My eyes swung from Dave to Andy; I thought this answer seemed a bit harsh. I was in hyperactive coddling mode, like a hovering mother, affirming and rewarding Dave for every little thing he did or attempted.

"We should correct him when he says things that make no sense," Andy said, looking from me to his parents and then back to Dave. "You *aren't* going to die, Dave; do you hear me? It's June 13, 2015, and you're in Chicago. You're at Rush. You had a stroke, but you're getting the best possible care and we're all here for you. We love you, Dave. You understand?"

It was fairly obvious that Dave did not understand what was going on, but we would keep telling him, as many times as we needed to, until hopefully he could.

❧ ❧ ❧

Dave could not swallow. That most life-sustaining and fundamental of bodily actions, coordinated between the brain and the muscles of the mouth and throat—an action automatically performed even by newborns in their first seconds of life on their mothers' breasts—was beyond Dave's brain. So he could not eat solid or even liquified food, but instead he continued to receive his nutrients through an IV. After a few days, once he did pass "the swallow test" (yes, that's a real thing), I was allowed to feed him gelatinous mounds of pureed mush. He could not hold the silverware for himself, so there he sat, wearing a bib and listening to orders to "open up," just like we had planned to do for our baby in a few months.

"This is turkey, your favorite," I said, my voice falsely chipper as I glanced from the menu card on the tray to the glob of beige jelly on the dinner plate. Most of his nutrients were still being delivered through the intravenous tube, one of the many wires snaking around his medical cot, connecting his pierced body to a constellation of hospital machines and screens. And though Dave could walk with assistance to the bathroom, he could not be trusted to know when he needed to *use* the bathroom, so he remained catheterized. Tubes in and tubes out—so many tubes performing the bodily functions that my husband was no longer able to perform for himself.

Due to the stroke's impact on Dave's cranial nerves, his eyes could not move from side to side or up and down. When he looked at me, he had to swivel his entire head to move his gaze, and he often had a blank and vacant expression, appearing confused or like he could not really see me. This, I would come to find out, was because *he could not really see me.* Dave was seeing everything in double vision. He appeared confused because he *was* confused, but he did not have the words to tell us.

All of this—the vacant stare, the mangled and incoherent

words, the wires and the machines and the accidents in bed—combined to form a whole picture that could not have looked less like my husband. Dave was there physically, yes. And yet the question I asked myself in silence—my heart aching in my chest, my mind spinning in panic—was this: *who was this man, really, if Dave's mind no longer occupied this broken body?*

The doctors came in and out in an endless procession, crisp white coats and firm handshakes and so many questions about Dave's habits and behavior and any other significant detail we might have overlooked—anything that might break open the mystery of this rare and confounding stroke. I struggled to remember the flurry of names and titles and roles. What I *do* remember is feeling like we had to pass a big test each time they appeared and asked Dave the litany of questions. *What's your name? Where are you? Why are you here? What's the date?*

When Dave's neurologist told him that we were in Chicago and then, a minute later, Dave could not answer the question "Where are you?," a sinking feeling settled in. It was all so odd; Dave could tell us that George W. Bush had been in Delta Kappa Epsilon, Dave's college fraternity, but he could not tell us where he was or why he was there or what year it was.

At night, after Dave had gone to sleep, I would open my laptop and continue my nightly ritual of writing to my husband. I did not want to leave Dave. I did not want to go home yet—back to our silent, empty apartment, where photos of a smiling, strong Dave looked at me from the walls. Where our dog would greet me at the door, tail wagging, before sniffing around for the other half of her family.

I would watch Dave sleep in his hospital bed and I would type. With the ever-present rhythmic beeping of the hospital machines as my accompaniment, I would rehash the day, typing in a stream of consciousness about what Dave had done and who had visited. I did not count on myself to remember all of the intense and emotionally charged moments of these long ICU days, and I knew for certain that there was no way Dave would ever remember them, and yet a part of me wanted to believe that, someday, Dave would be alert and interested enough to know about these moments he was living. This nightmare we were living.

The laptop perched on my legs, balanced in front of my swollen belly, I typed:

Dear Dave,

I'm so very sad. My thoughts had been on getting you stable enough to get you home to Chicago. Now that we're here . . . now what? Now what are we working for? The uncertainty is the worst part. I miss you so much, and no one can tell me with any certainty if you will ever come back to me. This is the worst pain I could have possibly imagined. I just really miss you.

We hoped that pieces of Dave were still in there, perhaps rendered unavailable and temporarily misplaced due to the stroke but still somewhat intact, and so we did everything we could to stimulate his brain and trigger his memories. I covered the hospital room with photos—shots from our wedding day, the most recent ultrasound images of the baby, pictures of his brothers and nieces and nephews and of him playing sports. I played his favorite music. His friend Russell sent a digital picture frame loaded with images collected from many of our friends. Andy and Nelson spent hours copying old home videos onto a small handheld video player that Dave could watch in his hospital bed. I brought in banners and memorabilia from Dave's summer camp, high school football team, and college lacrosse team. I had his co-residents send the video of a roast Dave had cowritten about a bunch of their fellow residents the year earlier.

In those first few days, the medical team was hard at work trying to identify why the stroke had happened. Through an endless series of cardiograms, MRIs, and other tests, we determined that Dave's stroke was as improbable as we had initially thought in Fargo. Dave's anatomy and a handful of unique situational circumstances had amounted to the world's worst lottery ticket. To start with, Dave must have had a clot form in his leg. This alone was not entirely surprising; he had been sitting at his desk working on research literally all day for weeks. Or perhaps it was from sitting still on the plane.

This clot must have then traveled up from his leg to his heart. That, also, was not entirely shocking, as clots tend to travel in the bloodstream and will sometimes move toward the heart.

But there, something else happened. The doctors observed that Dave had what is known as a patent foramen ovale (PFO) in his heart. A relatively common condition believed to occur in approximately a quarter of all healthy adults, it's a small hole between the two atria of the heart, something that all babies are born with. This hole exists in all of us in the womb so that nutrient-rich blood can flow freely through our heart chambers before our own lungs perform the job of moving that blood for us. The hole typically closes on its own after birth. But Dave's PFO never closed. That is something he had not known about himself; it's something he really had not *needed* to know, as is the case with the roughly 25 to 30 percent of adults who are walking around with the same condition unaware. A PFO is not something that, on its own, is going to cause a healthy adult to have a stroke or any other major health crisis.

And yet, Dave's PFO likely led to the next nightmarish sequence of events. Without a PFO, a clot would normally go from the legs to the right atrium of the heart, then to the right ventricle and into the lungs, where, unless it was quite large, it would cause little harm. Unfortunately, at the instant that Dave's clot reached the right atrium, he must have done something to increase the right atrial pressure (cough, or more likely, lift our suitcases overhead on the plane), so the clot traveled into the left atrium, then the left ventricle and into the aorta. From there it could then have gone into any artery, the blockage not posing a serious danger.

But then, something even *more* unlikely occurred. The MRI results revealed that Dave has a rare anatomic variant in his brain called an artery of Percheron. Think about this artery as a tree. Most of us have "trees" with hundreds of branches (small arteries) feeding oxygen to the thalamic portion of the brain. When you have an artery of Percheron, however, rather than having all of those little branches, you just have one big trunk. This clot in most people would not be a problem; oxygen would still feed to both the right and left thalami through the many other branches, or arteries. But if you have just the one trunk, the one artery, then a clot means the entire passage is blocked. The oxygen flow is obstructed, and the brain's cells are starved of critical oxygen. This means a lot of dead and damaged neurons in the midbrain. So when Dave had turned to me on the plane to ask whether his eye looked weird, his brain had literally been in the process of suffocating.

If it sounds complicated and unlikely, it is because *it's extremely complicated and unlikely*. It's also very bad. It baffled the doctors and Nelson and Andy for days until they were able to cobble together the pieces of this complex and improbable puzzle—and the picture this finished puzzle formed was grim. That Dave had survived was—without a doubt—miraculous.

I tried my best to absorb this deluge of medical information, but rather than getting too far into the weeds with all of the science (I knew that his neurologist father and his cardiologist brother were poring over echocardiograms and MRIs and the medical literature), I focused on what Dave needed from me and what I was uniquely able to give him as his wife.

And I focused on my own grim truths. Dave would survive, but how would he live? His mind and body were decimated. Our world had fallen apart, and I had no idea how to piece it back to-gether—or what it could even look like if and when I did piece it back together.

And so, though Dave hadn't died, though I wasn't a widow at the age of thirty, though I wasn't planning a funeral and grieving the premature death of the love of my life, I *was* grieving. The Dave I had known and loved, the Dave I had married, the Dave I had planned to have a baby with—that man was no more. My Dave had looked at me on that plane with a dilated eye before slipping from consciousness; a different man had awoken in that hospital bed. A foreign man who looked at me with vacant, con-fused eyes. A man who could not remember his name, or the fact that we were having a baby together.

The life for which we had planned and hoped and worked— the life we had lived prior to nine P.M. on June 9—was gone. Those versions of Alli and Dave, the two people who had loved and lived in that life, they, too, were gone.

Our future, along with our present, and even our past, had been snatched suddenly and ingloriously away. And so I was mourning, in my own way. I was mourning the husband who was no longer there. And I was mourning the old version of myself, too. The version of myself who had boarded that plane; the ver-sion of myself who had stared boldly and confidently at our fu-ture; the version of myself who had had her Dave beside her, who had been happy and lucky and innocent.

I noticed absentmindedly as I looked out the window that it rained a lot—we were having an unseasonably wet June. *Good*, I thought, *I'm glad it is a bad June.* At least it seemed like Mother Nature was acknowledging the way I felt and mirroring it back to me. Beautiful sunny days might make it all the more painful, might remind me that other people were out in the world, enjoy-ing this favorite time of year. Just like I would have done, in a different life. In the life I might have had, had the stroke not happened.

Along those same lines of thinking, I flatly forbade myself from logging in to any sort of social media. As an author, one of the primary ways that I connect with readers and bloggers and fellow writers is via social media. I use it in my personal life as well. But I knew that, for the time being, it was a bad idea. It was summer, and people were bound to be enjoying vacations and barbecues, swimming in picturesque bodies of water, savoring the warm weather.

The last thing I needed was to log in to Instagram or Facebook and see a stream of glossy, edited photos of happy people eating lobster on a dock or drinking rosé in front of a beautiful sunset. Social media is bad enough for the mood and the self-esteem on a good day, when all we see is an endless sequence of people's highlight reels. I certainly did not need to see that and compare it to my view from the ICU. Social media is a siren call, with its ability to numb and distract, to pull us out of our own present and into the fabricated, filtered worlds of others. But as much as I did want to be pulled out of my world, as much as I did crave even just a few minutes of anything other than my reality—I had to forbid myself. I knew that, for the time being, I had to just remain still in that painful place, unpleasant as it was, as tempting as it was to seek some temporary diversion. I guessed that, in the end, the diversion would only make me feel worse. And the pain would remain. So I had to choose instead to stay in my painful present, where my focus and my energy were needed.

But man, was it difficult to be in that present. "This is especially hard for you because you like to have a plan. You like to feel in control," my mom said to me in those early days. "But there's nothing you can do here to plan or control the outcome. You just have to be with Dave. Just take it a day at a time, sweetie. Dave is strong, Alli, and he will fight as hard as he can. You just need to be here beside him right now."

I learned from the neuro-ICU nurses and doctors how to best stimulate and orient Dave. I repeated every few minutes where we were and why we were there. I fed him his food and talked to him about our baby. Several times a day I would try to motivate Dave for a big "outing"—we would walk a lap around the hospital floor, eyes fixed forward, not turning to look from left to right into the many other hospital rooms where so many other families were quietly engaged in their own agonies, their own life-and-death battles. My strong, athletic husband would lean on a walker, slowly shuffling forward as I walked beside him and a nurse trailed behind, a harness wrapped around his hospital gown to catch him when he wobbled. I monitored his bathroom visits and made sure he was staying hydrated. I filled out paperwork and spoke with doctors and befriended nurses and learned about his meds.

Like the countless other spouses and family members who have kept vigil beside the hospital bed of a loved one, I put everything else out of my mind and made that hospital room my entire world.

Dear Dave,
*   Before your cardiac test you looked scared. I asked you*
if you were scared and you nodded, so I took your hand and
told you where we were and that we were all here with you
and that you were going to get better. I love you so much.

Dave may not have known where he was or why he was there, but I would do my best to make sure that he knew he was not alone.

Chapter 15

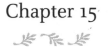

Dear Dave,
    I will meet many guardian angels along this journey.
I met one today.

I wrote that in my DearDave Word document on our first day at Rush. It was true; from the Fargo ICU to the Rush ICU, to rehab and beyond, strangers and loved ones emerged to walk beside us and help us forward through the crisis. One of the first angels we met was at Rush, and his name was Omar.

Dr. Omar Lateef was a specialist in pulmonary and critical care medicine, and now served as the chief medical officer at Rush University Medical Center. I remember, that first day, we kept hearing from our resident and attending physicians about some guy named Omar.

"Omar is on his way in."
"Omar is at home with his family, but he's driving in from the suburbs."
"You have to meet Omar; he really wants to talk to you."

So, our whole family sat down in a private conference room and we met Omar.

From that first day at Rush, Omar took Dave—and all of us—under his wing. We did not know it from Fargo, but Omar had had his hand in everything from facilitating the air ambulance ride to getting Dave a room at Rush on the neuro-ICU floor. Omar reserved the family conference room where we could congregate and where the young niece and nephews (who were not allowed onto the floor of the neuro-ICU) could gather and run around and nap. Omar had a tray of sandwiches waiting for us at dinnertime. When the national press began to sniff around the hospital, hoping for a photo from the ER, Omar added security and made sure that our privacy was protected. Omar ensured that all of Dave's paperwork was done quickly and that all the parties from the Fargo ER to the Rush cardiology department to the insurance companies were working fluidly and efficiently together. As he does for each one of his patients, Omar worked to get Dave the best possible care and all the tests he needed as quickly as they were medically advisable.

At one point Omar took me aside. "Do you have out-of-town family? Friends? I know that if my wife were in your situation, she would need her mom with her. There's just something about her with her mom—it's like some secret language I can't understand. So you make sure you have whomever you need with you here. Does anyone need a hotel room?" Omar then pulled out his personal credit card, and I realized that he was offering to book the hotel room for us. The man's generosity was automatic, unthinking. "Anything we can do for you guys, you are family. Dave is one of our own."

Even just thinking about it now makes me want to cry all over again. Especially touching was how available Omar made himself as a friend and confidant, approachable in spite of his busy schedule and his demanding role as a leader at the hospital. His style was a special and rare blend of compassion and understanding mixed with irreverent humor and stubborn hope. A husband, a father of three, a doctor, and a significant figure in the hospital administration, Omar somehow knew every patient by name. Even more remarkable, he knew each patient's *family members* by name. He commented on my brother-in-law Mike's new hair-cut! I truly do not know when the guy slept or ate; he would check in at all hours. He would stop by the hospital room and pull me out and give me pep talks when he could read the fatigue and sadness and worry on my face after a long day.

Omar gave us hope when there was very little reason to cling to any. He believed that Dave's brain could heal, and that Dave's recovery could be nothing short of our wildest hopes. "This is all so new and shocking to you, but let me tell you: we see this all the time." There was something deeply reassuring about hearing that from Omar. It was not some platitude or cliché coming from someone who, though well meaning, really did not know what they were talking about. Omar knew what he was talking about. It *was* all so new and shocking to me. I could not believe any of it was happening. But to hear that Omar and his doctors had seen other people go through experiences this earth-shattering—to hear that people could survive and even recover—that normal-ized it a bit.

"And when this is all over, you and Dave are going to take me and my wife out for dinner, OK? You'll leave the baby at home, because it's impossible to enjoy a restaurant with the kids, wait and you'll see. So, no kids. How do cheeseburgers sound?" Omar smiled and I agreed. "It's a deal."

I remember something else Omar said in the very beginning. He was speaking to me as a friend rather than a doctor, and he told me: "Pray. Pray to whatever deity you believe in, or ask the universe, or meditate—however you think of prayer. I really be-lieve it helps in ways we can't explain."

Once, when Omar went far out on a limb to help us in an insurance dispute that could have been catastrophic had it not gone our way, I asked him: "Why are you helping us so much? As busy as you are, how can you possibly devote this much time and energy and care to our *one* case like this?"

"Because I believe it's the right thing to do, not only as a doctor, but as a human being," Omar told me. "And I believe in God, so I want to do God's work. I want to do the right thing for people."

The topic of faith and prayer had come up in various ways in my conversations with Omar, and so finally one day I asked him the question that had been on my mind: "You talk about prayer and faith a lot, and I agree with you. What faith do you practice?" Whatever his faith walk was, I wanted to know, because I admired it. Omar was walking the walk of God's love every single day of his life.

Omar told me that he had studied many different religions, and had even focused on theology as part of his schooling, but he himself identified as Muslim. So there we were, a Muslim and a Christian, sitting in the hospital room talking about faith and medicine, both of us pulling for Dave with the best resources we could bring to the difficult situation. I do not know if Omar was aware that he was treating not only Dave but Dave's whole family.

All we could do at that point was fumble in the darkness of our fear and the unknown, but the support coming from Omar and others provided the shards of light that we needed in order to keep moving forward, one faltering step at a time.

So many of the words of comfort we would hear in those early days would come in the form of well-worn clichés:

> *"It's a marathon, not a sprint."*
> *"Take it day by day."*
> *"It'll be a long road."*

*"It will be a roller coaster; you have to take the highs
   with the lows."*
"Two steps forward, one step backward."

As tiresome as it could be to hear these pat turns of phrase,
there was a certain wisdom in their age-old truths. It *would* be a
long road. It *would* be a marathon—but I could not really understand any of that right then. At that point we were still very much
in the "sprint" phase. I was not thinking about conserving energy
or digging in for the long haul, bracing myself for the cruel roller
coaster that is traumatic brain injury. I was thinking about spending every minute with Dave and putting every drop of energy I
had into his treatment and recovery. Telling him, hour after hour,
where he was and that he was going to get better.

Did I truly believe, in the private places of my own heart, that
Dave would in fact get better? I didn't know. I am an information
junkie and I like to study and seek answers, but in this situation,
perhaps the hardest part was that there were no answers. Control
was an illusion that had been shattered into a million tiny pieces
the moment Dave lost consciousness on that plane.

We received so many notes of support in those early days, but
there was one in particular that provided a lifeline for me. Lee
Woodruff, married to ABC News anchor Bob Woodruff, had been
through her own life-changing experience as the partner and
caregiver to a traumatic-brain-injury patient. Bob nearly lost his
life when his convoy drove over a roadside bomb while covering
the Iraq War in 2006. I had gotten to know Lee a little over the
years, first when I was working at ABC News, and then in the
writing world we shared as authors in the New York area. Lee had
reached out after the stroke through my sister, Emily, gently making herself available to talk—an open invitation with no pressure
or expectations attached.

One Sunday night, I took Lee up on the offer. Dave was asleep in his ICU bed, and I did not have an apartment to go home to because we were in the process of moving and my whole bedroom was packed in boxes and bubble wrap. I was crashing on a friend's couch for a couple of days. Curled up on that couch, I dialed Lee and I wept. We talked about how the phrase "Everything happens for a reason" fell painfully flat. We spoke about how scared I was to have a baby—I didn't know how I could possibly take care of Dave and a newborn. We spoke about how unfair it all felt. We spoke about how the many unknowns were the cruelest part. Lee promised me that it would get better, somehow, some way.

"I know you can't possibly see it right now, because it's so new and horrible and it's so scary, but I can promise you two things. Number one, it will be different. Life has changed, life will forever be different. But here's number two: even though it will be different, it *will* be OK," Lee said. "I promise you, somehow, it will be OK."

I didn't see how she could be correct, but I clung to her words. She was, after all, speaking with the insight and understanding of someone who had walked a path similar to my own. Someone who had scaled a similarly grueling peak and had made it to the summit, where things did begin to look manageable—albeit entirely altered—once more.

"Life will never look exactly the same as it did before. But as my Bob tells me: Who knows what it would have looked like and who would ever believe it could be perfect? What is perfect anyway? And who cares now? Those imaginary visions are only a film torture loop. Turn off the movie in your head called *My Once and Glorious Life.* We don't get to take that particular footpath now. That one got shut down by an avalanche. As soon as we accept the fact that we got rerouted, we can move forward into the world with all the tools and love and friends and grace and hope and faith and beauty that we just got reminded are ours."

I absorbed these words—crying and nodding. They brought both pain and hope. At one point, I asked: "Why are you doing this, Lee?" It was a Sunday night in early summer. Lee has four kids and a husband and a full career and a huge and happy life, and I could not believe she was taking an hour to talk to some weeping person she'd only met a couple of times in passing. "Why are you making this time for me?"

"I'm doing this because, though you might not believe me right now, someday your life will be good again. And someday, years from now, someone will need to hear from you about this moment. And so you'll find yourself sitting on the couch at home on a Sunday night, speaking to someone who needs you, and you'll tell this person that they can get through whatever it is that they are going through. That's all part of the deal, OK?"

I agreed.

Lee said: "I am here as your friend to welcome you to the 'Club of the Bad Thing.'"

It was a club I wanted no part of. Of course I wanted no part of it. Who would? But, there I was. And then, thinking back to Dave's playlist of classic rock, the one I had played in the emergency room that first night in Fargo, I began to hear the tune to the Eagles' hit "Hotel California." *You can check out anytime you like, but you can never leave.*

Chapter 16

Paris, France
May 2010

ON MY FIRST DAY IN PARIS I IGNORED THE JET LAG AND I
walked all the way from the sixteenth arrondissement, just north-
west of Avenue Foch, past the Arc de Triomphe, down the Champs-
Élysées, through Place de la Concorde, past the Louvre Museum
and the Tuileries Garden, across Île de la Cité and Île Saint-Louis
and over to the Left Bank. There, sitting on the terrace of a café
eating a late lunch, overlooking the Seine and Bateaux Mouches
boats that glided by, gawking at the gargoyle spires of Notre
Dame in the near distance, I could not believe that I had done it.
I had quit my very sensible job writing daytime news and had left
my New York City apartment in the hands of a subletter and had
relocated, alone, to Paris.

And not just Paris, but Paris in the full and rapturous throes of
springtime. The chestnut and plane trees hung heavy with new
leaves along the riverside quays; adorable little children squealed

with delight as they skipped across cobblestones on their way home from school. From where I was sitting, I could hear an accordion. I could hear fragments of French as people passed by. I could hear the peals of Notre Dame's bells. On my walk home, I could stop at any number of bakeries and get myself an oven-fresh *pain au chocolat,* the gooey inside still warm and liquid. My soul was dancing for joy.

Dave had fully supported my decision. He had seen better than anyone how deeply I had longed to make a career change. He was finishing up an intense period of medical school and was busy himself. I would be back in New York City in the fall.

I saw my time in Paris, my favorite city in the world, as a chance to replenish my soul. After feeling stressed, overstimulated, and unfulfilled during the years working a job that was not the right fit, Paris was a chance to make a meaningful shift. It was time to be by myself and contemplate what I wanted for these next steps in my life and in my career and in my relationship with Dave. It was, as I saw it, a last opportunity to go off on my own and have adventures and live according to my whims in a rich and beautiful and transient moment.

I do not mind traveling alone. In fact, I love traveling alone. I bought a Europass, and I took the train all over Europe that spring. I visited family friends in glorious Florence and then took the bus through Tuscany and visited Siena. I went to Geneva to stay with my aunt Tessa, whose Parisian apartment I was occupying, and we rode a chairlift across stunning Alpine vistas and climbed old church bell towers. I met my friend Charlotte in Bruges, Belgium, and we traveled together to her family's hometown on the coast of the North Sea in Ostend, Belgium, where we ate *frites* and drank Belgian beer and meandered through the markets and squares. I traveled throughout France, visiting the medieval walled city of Saint-Malo and the Breton coast (where my mother's family originally came from) and capping off a wonderful *séjour* with my cousin's beautiful wedding at her family home in Plouër-sur-Rance.

I remember, one afternoon in Florence, I was walking around the city, several generous scoops of gelato balancing atop a cone in my hand. I was devouring the ice cream; I was devouring the views of that magical city. I was savoring my freedom and the sounds of the church bells and the snippets of Italian and the wonder of it all. I passed shops and kiosks and wound my way through narrow cobblestoned streets, enjoying myself without a map or an agenda. As I ambled across the magnificent Piazza del Duomo, one of the store owners raised his arms, proclaiming: *"Bella signorina,* you look happy!"

I smiled and answered: "I am."

Chapter 17

"PLASTIC." I'D NEVER KNOWN IT WAS A WORD THAT COULD DE-scribe a human brain, but it was something we heard all the time in those early days and weeks after the stroke. "Neuronal plasticity." A cursory Internet search will tell you that neuronal plasticity is "the brain's ability to reorganize itself by forming new neural connections throughout life. Neuroplasticity allows the neurons (nerve cells) in the brain to compensate for injury and disease and to adjust their activities in response to new situations or to changes in their environment."

Sizable portions of Dave's brain were dead, wiped out from not having received oxygen. Neuronal plasticity would be Dave's best hope for recovery. Neuronal plasticity became our buzzword, our lifeline, our mantra, and our hope. All brains have this plastic quality, which is why even Alzheimer's patients in their eighties can and should work to stimulate their brain's functionality. We are all encouraged to do things to facilitate plasticity, even something as simple as brushing your teeth with your nondominant hand or taking a shower with your eyes shut. New experiences and challenges force us to get out of our automatic routines and encourage the brain to form new neuronal pathways, thereby staying active and agile.

The brain is the most remarkable and least understood organ in the body, and its ability to regenerate and evolve defies scientific understanding. But here's the thing: neuronal plasticity, that nebulous characteristic that allows for "miracles" in victims of traumatic brain injury, changes over the course of a life. A huge part of plasticity is related to age. Newborns are incredibly plastic. Anyone who has ever observed a baby knows this to be true: their brains change very quickly, on a daily basis as they learn and grow. Plasticity decreases with age, so the older you are, the less plastic your brain is. The cutoff for when this neuronal plasticity begins to decrease? Around age thirty to thirty-five. Dave was thirty years old.

If Dave had had this stroke even one year later, his hopes for recovery might have been significantly reduced. If he had had this stroke five years later, he very likely would not have survived. At thirty, Dave had youth—and more neuronal plasticity—on his side, and that helped his chances of recovery.

We needed this plasticity because while my husband was there physically, he was still not there mentally. As we checked days off the calendar, Dave still did not know where he was, even though it was the hospital in which he had spent every single day for the previous three years. What was especially heartbreaking to me was that Dave did not remember that we had a beloved black mutt named Penny. Dave and that dog were madly in love; the last thing we had done together before getting on the plane was look at photos of her. At one point, he told me we had a cat (we've never had a cat). At other times he told me we had a yellow Lab or that her name was Xena, who had been his childhood dog.

On Monday, June 15, the rain was absolutely apocalyptic over Chicago. My mother, who was staying with me for a couple of weeks, drove me home from the hospital, and we thought we were going to get stuck in the flooding. The voice on the radio informed us that there had been a tornado outside Chicago earlier that day. "I hope the game doesn't get canceled," I said. Dave's favorite hockey team, the Chicago Blackhawks, was playing to win the Stanley Cup that night.

Dave watched from his bed in the ICU with Brad, one of his best friends, as I headed home after a long day. The Blackhawks won. The old Dave would have been so happy. He had followed the whole season and postseason with a giddy hope. He had planned to watch the championship games in Hawaii. I would not have cared, to be honest. In that alternate life, given the time difference, I probably would have been outside reading by the ocean and would have come inside to Dave's smile and happy proclamation that his team had won. I would have been happy that he was happy, but I would not have been *moved.*

But that was in the alternate life. The one that was no longer going to happen. In *this* life, I cared. I watched every minute of the game that night in Dave's honor, deeply invested. When they won, I wept. Dave's friend Russell texted me, elated: "**That was for Dave!**"

Our apartment faced west, looking out over the Chicago River and the western suburbs. I stood before the window and stared out; I could see Rush in the distance, where Dave was, across the flat Midwestern landscape. I could see, not too far from Rush, the United Center, where the Blackhawks had just won hockey's highest honor. Fireworks burst across the sky. All of Chicago was celebrating as I stood at the window and wept.

The next morning when I arrived at Dave's hospital room, he did not remember that the Blackhawks had won. He did not remember that he'd watched, that Brad had come for the game and that they'd sat together and eaten pizza and that his favorite player, Patrick Kane, had scored the game-winning goal.

The letters I wrote to Dave at the end of each day became all the more important. If he came back, he could read these letters and understand what he had gone through. *If* he came back. God, it hurt. If he came back. I loved so many things about Dave, but, most of all, I loved his brain. I loved his mind. I loved his wit. That, over the years, we had developed our own shorthand of inside jokes and code words and shared experiences. These were the things that made Dave mine. That was what made this injury so completely devastating: an arm, I could do without. But his mind? How could I live without Dave's mind?

Dear Dave,
    I need to be patient. I just miss you so much.

Chapter 18

Adirondack State Park, New York
August 2010

I suspected that Dave was about to pop the question. It was the end of the summer, and I had just moved back from Paris to New York. In a month, Dave was to start an independent research year between his third and fourth years of medical school.

Dave's parents were flying out to join us at my parents' place in upstate New York, where we have a family farm on Lake Champlain. I thought Dave might propose that week, with both sets of family there and the peaceful, natural setting as a backdrop. The reason Dave was taking a research year was so that he could have a period with a more manageable workload between seven straight years of schooling, and for both of us to catch our breaths before he began applying to residency programs. I'd quit news, and we were both taking steps to find more happiness in our day-to-day lives, specifically on the work front, and we had decided to make our relationship a higher priority. The timing felt right.

The morning Dave's parents were scheduled to arrive, he and I sat by the lake, just the two of us. I had my feet dangling off the dock, the view of Vermont's Green Mountains spanning the scene before us.

Dave turned to me and said, casual as could be: "I guess I should get your ring size at some point."

I paused a moment, taken aback. "Wait, what?"

"Your ring size. If I'm going to propose at some point, I should know the size of your finger."

I looked out over the water, silenced. *Huh,* I thought, *so he is just now getting around to the thought of getting a ring. I guess it's not happening this week.*

I noticed the sinking feeling in my stomach. I'd questioned whether I was ready to get engaged, but here I was, disappointed. As it turned out, I *was* ready to marry Dave, more ready than I had thought.

That afternoon, after several flight delays and a ferry ride across Lake Champlain, Dave's parents arrived at our farm. While they settled in before dinner, Dave suggested he and I take a quick walk with the dogs. We headed away from the lake and the house, meandering up the hill to a field carpeted in clover. My mom had told us that it was a great place to scout for four-leaf clovers. All that week Dave had been on the lookout for a four-leaf clover, but so far neither of us had had any luck in finding one.

I paused to scan the view from this hill. It was the predinner hour, and upstate New York was awash in gentle summer sunshine. Before us stretched rural green fields that met Lake Champlain, and beyond that, on the other shore, layers of Vermont's stunning mountains. There was no point in taking a photo, because no photo could have fully captured the beauty of the moment.

"Look, a four-leaf clover!" Dave bent over as we crested the hill. I followed his pointing.

"I don't see it," I said, but then I looked at him. He was on one knee, and he was holding—to my surprise—a ring. He told me that he couldn't imagine life without me. He called me by the series of nicknames he had used over our six years together. I cried, my hands trembling as Dave slid the ring on my finger—a ring he'd designed to look like my grandmother's, because I had told him years ago that I loved my grandmother's ring. We sat together on the hilltop and looked out over the lake and joined hands to offer up a prayer of thanksgiving.

When we returned to the house, there was champagne and hugging and ogling of the ring. It was all so sickeningly sweet.

The next day, on a walk with our families, Dave and I found three four-leaf clovers.

We were giddy—we'd never found one before that day, and now suddenly we had three. We took it as a propitious sign.

We kept those clovers. I pressed them and glued them to a photo of us. The photo was taken by Dave's dad on the afternoon of that walk, right when we found those clovers. In it Dave and I stand side by side, beaming, glowing from our suntans and the excitement of the engagement, still less than twenty-four hours old at that point.

I wrote a note on that photo, right beneath the pressed clovers:

Dear Dave,
*   May we always remember how "lucky" we are*
to have one another—
*   Love,*
*   Alli*

At my bridal shower three months before our wedding, my godmother gave me a necklace with a silver four-leaf clover, in honor of our story. On the night before we got married, my mother-in-law told everyone this story at the rehearsal dinner.

When I looked at the man seated beside me, holding my hand through the evening of toasts, I wanted to bottle it all up, save it, carry it with us into our future together.

May we always remember how lucky we are. I gave that photo with those clovers as a gift to Dave on our wedding day. I'd written that caption because I knew, even then, that in spite of how much we loved each other, in spite of the fact that we were so happy to be marrying each other, that there would be days when we would forget the good fortune that had brought us together. We would have days when we took our lives and our love for granted. When we failed to give thanks for our many blessings and would need a reminder. I knew that, even with that message hanging on our wall, there would be days when we would forget, and that on those days, we would need to remember.

Chapter 19

TIMING IS SO IMPORTANT IN THE RECOVERY AFTER A TRAU-
matic brain injury. On the one hand, every neurologist will tell
you that "it is going to take time." And yet, you want to work
quickly, as it's a race to recapture as much as you can as quickly
as you can while the brain is still in a state of healing. Time becomes this shifty entity, at once both ally and enemy.

Once Dave was medically stable and the threat of a repeat
event was ruled out, his team agreed that it was important to get
him into an inpatient rehabilitation facility where he could get
right to work on rebuilding and replacing and reconnecting those
dead and damaged neurons. We considered a few options, but
really the answer was clear to us all from the beginning—for recovery, Dave would go to the Rehabilitation Institute of Chicago,
ranked the nation's number one rehabilitation center for more
than twenty consecutive years. It was incredibly fortuitous that
such world-class rehabilitation existed in our city, ten minutes
from our apartment.

As thrilled as I was to be getting out of the frenetic, sterile,
nerve-addling ICU, I was anxious about the transition to a place

where we would have a lot more autonomy; I was reluctant to be giving up the round-the-clock medical care and monitoring that made the hospital both a blessing and a curse. I worried that the care these expert ICU nurses had been providing would fall largely on my shoulders. I worried that I would forget when Dave had to take his medication or that I wouldn't know what to do in case of an emergency. A task as simple as shaving confounded me—Dave was in no way capable of handling a razor, so who would shave his face?

Most intimidating to me was the daily monitoring of Dave's heart. Since the stroke, Dave had been wearing a heart monitor. We suspected that the PFO (the hole in Dave's heart) had played a part in the circumstances that led to the stroke, and Dave's cardiologist wanted to be sure that there was not a larger problem like an arrhythmia (irregular heartbeat) or another possible congenital heart deformity. Dave was to wear the monitor for a month, and the electrodes had to be changed each night before bed. They were red and black and white and had to correspond to particular wires and particular places on Dave's chest. The battery had to be charged each night and replaced each day. The monitor communicated with a recording device, much like a cellphone, that had to be within ten feet of Dave at all times. In the more mobile setting of rehab, where Dave was shuffling from room to room for various therapy treatments, this would mean the device would have to go everywhere with him. Dave was in no way capable of remembering something like this, so it fell on me. I brought a pouch from home that Dave could wear around his neck each day with this small heart monitor inside, much like a tourist would wear to keep money safe while traveling in a foreign country. I cannot tell you how many times I trailed behind him, waving that pouch like a mother brandishing her kid's forgotten homework as the school bus pulls away: "You forgot your heart monitor! Put your pouch around your neck!"

Dave and I went together in the ambulance from Rush to RIC. He was still in a state of complete amnesia, and so even though I tried to explain the situation to him, he did not understand why we were in an ambulance. Strapped into a wheelchair, leg and arm restraints in place to ensure he would not get up, Dave panicked. He kept trying to break free from the straps, and, given his strength, he was coming perilously close to doing just that. He kept reaching for the door of the ambulance to open it.

"What are you doing?" I asked, my voice growing shrill. It was just Dave and me in the back of that ambulance, and I would not be able to restrain him if he managed to wriggle free.

"I don't want to be here. I want to go home," Dave told me, looking distrustfully around the inside of the ambulance.

"I know you do, and we will go home soon, I promise. But first we have to go to rehab. We are going together; I will be with you. It's the best rehab facility in the country, and we will be in the best hands possible."

Though I had told him this a dozen times, Dave looked at me now, trying to understand this information. He shook his head and began a fresh round of writhing and squirming, his hands working to undo the straps that were barely holding him in place. "No, I want to go home."

Trust me, so do I, I thought. We were on the highway in rush-hour traffic. I was six months pregnant. What would I do if I had to physically restrain my husband, who weighed almost twice what I did? How would I keep him from opening the door and jumping out onto the highway?

"What do I do?" I asked the driver, my panic rising by the second as my husband thrashed and jerked around in the wheel-chair. The driver was on his cellphone, speaking to a friend in colorful language about the physical attributes of a lady friend of his. He did not seem to hear my desperate entreaties. He kept chatting away as Dave kept writhing and fighting against his restraint straps. *Please please please just let us get there,* I thought. The whole situation was so absurd that I wanted to laugh and cry at the same time.

Finally, after contending with the traffic jams, we made it, pulling up in front of RIC with Dave still fastened in his wheelchair. I told him for the twentieth time where we were and why we were there. I told him he was at RIC to get the best rehab treatment in the world.

As we settled Dave into his room, I looked around at our new home base. As a nurse reviewed the inpatient information with us, a middle-aged woman, another inpatient, wandered into our room, clearly disoriented. A moment later a kind nurse came in and guided her out. "We don't go into other people's rooms," the nurse said gently as they walked away. I slid the curtain across the room's entrance, trying to gain some privacy for us. I looked back toward Dave, and around at our room.

As we sat there, the extent of Dave's handicaps settled in my gut with a harsh new clarity. The bed restraints, the wheelchair that they were insisting Dave use anytime he left his room, the safeguards in the bathroom. How depressing would all of this be for Dave if and when he realized just how incapacitated he was? How would day after day in this sterile, hospital-like environment cause him to feel anything other than utter despair? He was supposed to be working as a doctor, operating on people at that very moment, living a full and vibrant life as a healthy thirty-year-old with a wife and a baby on the way, and, instead, he was the youngest person (by decades) on a floor filled with people who were either physically or mentally incapacitated. How damn unlucky was he?

This is something I have never shared—not even with my mother-in-law, or my mother, or even with Dave. In that moment, I looked around the space with even wider eyes; I looked with horror at the hooks on the ceiling, from which they secure safety straps for people who can't walk. I had the horrific, blood-chilling thought: *What if Dave tries to hang himself?*

Unpacking there, though trying to remain outwardly upbeat for Dave, I had a feeling similar to the one I'd had when we first arrived at the Rush ICU. In Fargo, I had been looking ahead to getting Dave back to Chicago because it would mean he was stable enough to travel and it would mean getting home, back to loved ones and familiar territory and Rush's world-class neurology ICU. Then at Rush I had been looking ahead to getting Dave to RIC because it would mean he was medically strong enough that we could stop worrying about him dying, and we could focus on his getting better. We could start the work of bringing his brain back online.

But here we were. Settled in at RIC. Now what? Dave's amnesia and helplessness were still our reality. There was nowhere else to go, nowhere else to be but in that dreadful reality.

Chapter 20

Hudson Valley, New York
September 2011

I WAS TOLD SO MANY TIMES THINGS LIKE "YOUR WEDDING will be a blur," "You won't remember a thing," and "It will go by so quickly, it'll be over before you know it," that I made a concerted effort not to allow the weekend to go by in a blur. The yogi in me worked hard to "be present" for all of it, and our wedding was quite a bash.

It was funny how Dave had strong opinions about just a few, very specific things: the texture of the bread during the dinner (I'm not kidding, the man takes his bread very seriously, and he did not want the rolls to be *too* crispy), the forks we registered for (as he said, "We'll be eating off these forks for the rest of our lives, it's important we get this right"), the seating arrangements, and a few other things. He sweetly requested that I wear at least some of my hair down as opposed to an upswept look because that is how he prefers it normally. But other than that, he let me and my mother run with most of the planning, and we did, and we had a blast doing it together.

There was one minor mishap a week before the wedding, when the stylist from the big, fancy New York City salon gave me "highlights" that turned out to be a single tone of platinum blond. I am a natural brunette with dark brown eyes; I can pull off natural highlights that fall somewhere in the family of "golden" or "honey," but this was "porn-star meets Playboy bunny," according to one rather honest friend. That, I could not pull off. Three appointments later, only after returning to the guy who had originally done my highlights as a teenager in upstate New York before I got all fancy, I got my hair back to some semblance of a naturally occurring color, albeit still a touch lighter than my original preference.

The wedding day itself went off without a hitch. The ceremony was in the local Catholic church and the party was in the backyard of my childhood home, where we danced all night surrounded by hundreds of loved ones. One of the primary reasons we had wanted to get married so close to home was because my grandmother, about to turn ninety-six, was largely housebound by that time. She had waited long enough for this day and there was no way I was going to let her miss it. For our wedding date Dave and I had chosen the same date on which Grandma and Grandpa had gotten married nearly three-quarters of a century earlier, and I wanted to make sure that she and I got our dance together.

My favorite part of the entire weekend was seeing Dave standing at the altar. We had not done a "first look" beforehand, so en vogue these days, and the church was the first place we saw each other on our wedding day. I remember feeling so nervous standing with my dad outside the door to the church in the moments before I walked down the aisle. My stomach felt like I had swallowed an entire bowl of goldfish as I watched my sister and sister-in-law and best friends process past in their gorgeous bridesmaid gowns.

And then, the "Wedding March" began to play, my dad led me inside, and I saw Dave. All the nerves—*poof!*—were gone in that instant. Our eyes locked. This was what it was all about. I was marrying this man. Everything else, everyone else, vanished. As I walked down the aisle, I saw Dave fighting back tears. "I couldn't believe it, that first glimpse I had," Dave told me later. "I couldn't believe that I was seeing you in a wedding dress and that you were walking towards me."

When the priest had asked us if we would be writing our own vows or saying traditional ones, we'd decided to go with the traditional. The writer in me believed that there was no way to top those age-old words, uttered on that happiest of days since time immemorial. What could be more powerful than the words "I, Allison, take you, David, for better or for worse, for richer or for poorer, in sickness and in health, for as long as we both shall live"?

I meant those words. I did. I did not just blindly recite them; it was a commitment I was thoughtfully and purposefully making. I'd put more thought into that decision than any other in my life. And I realized that all of those contingency clauses, the words like "in sickness and in health," would have their day of reckoning. I had seen both my grandmothers nurse my grandfathers at the ends of their lives. I knew that would happen to Dave and to me at some point. But as I stood there at the altar, I thought we were looking at, say, seventy years before that was upon us. "For as *long* as we both shall live." We would live a *long* time. At some point in the distant future, I would be required to summon fortitude and accept days that would not be fun, days of caregiving for an ailing and elderly spouse, or vice versa. At the end of a long and happy and full life, about the time our grandkids were making their own wedding vows—I would have a chance to live out the truth of these vows.

I had not realized that it would be so soon, on the near side of thirty.

But on that day we didn't think about any of that. When I look at pictures of us from our wedding I see only smiles of innocence and confidence and joy, two people so totally consumed in that present elation, a pair who think only with excitement about everything life will throw at them.

Chapter 21

SITTING IN ONE OF THE HOSPITAL ROOMS, DAVE ASLEEP IN THE bed between us, I confided something to my in-laws. "All my life," I said, "I've had this nagging fear that I was too lucky. That somehow, at some point, I would have to pay for the fact that I've been too lucky."

It was not the first time I had confessed this fatalistic fear. At Yale, one of the school traditions is the secret societies of senior year. You are "tapped" at the end of junior year to join a group with fifteen of your classmates. The group meets every week in a private home on campus, and one of the traditions is that each member of the group shares his or her "biography" with the group. This is the chance to bring everyone into the story of your past and to explain what, up until that point, has made you the person you are. Participating in it, we all felt very serious and self-important, naturally. During my "bio," I told the group that I worried that I had perhaps been too lucky—that I would eventually have to pay for the good fortune I'd so far enjoyed.

Specifically, I believed that I had been too lucky to have found Dave so early. Ours had been an easy love in the sense that it had been the easiest thing in the world to fall in love and, so far, it had been relatively easy to remain in love. That's not to say that our relationship was perfect. No, neither Dave nor I was perfect—far from it—and our relationship had its ups and downs just like all relationships do. But, so far, the moments of challenge or conflict had not proven insurmountable, and we had always come together to work through our differences. And so I felt like there was something I couldn't quite trust about it; people did not get this lucky in their love lives, not on the first real try. They did not get the happy ending without a whole bunch of heartbreak first. I felt that I was doomed to be dealt at least one big doozy. True, there had been that guy in high school where the affection had been weighted a little more on my side, and that had been painful at times, but it had not been a full-blown heartbreak. I was Dave's first serious girlfriend and he was my first deep and life-changing love—and here we were, still together. And having a baby! And here's the kicker: *I didn't even have morning sickness.* It hardly seemed fair.

At college, I'd had the privilege of taking a Shakespeare seminar with the legendary Harold Bloom. Professor Bloom had told us: "Make no mistake, you will all have your hearts broken at least once. Whether it's a lover or a child or a parent or a friend— somehow, your heart *will* be broken."

Up until that point, I was realizing, I had enjoyed a pretty charmed life, a life free of major heartbreak. Two supportive and loving parents, still alive and happily married. The same for Dave. His mother had gotten sick with multiple myeloma, and that had been excruciating and frightening, an earth-shaking trial for the entire family, but Louisa had made a miraculous comeback from a diagnosis that could have turned out to be far worse. She was strong once more, in remission, and so even in that, Dave and I had counted ourselves incredibly fortunate. What's more, we had close relationships with our siblings and plenty of wonderful friends. I loved my work as a writer; I felt like I got to wake up every morning and play make-believe—and I got paid to do it! I was young and healthy and in a marriage that was for the most part solid and happy, a bond forged in deep understanding and faithful commitment, in a shared history and significant experiences. There was no way to deny it: Dave and I had been remarkably lucky.

That was, until the stroke. As I confessed that fear to Louisa and Nelson, they both returned my gaze with knowing nods. They confessed that they, too, had had the same thought. For Dave and me, but also for themselves.

Now, from our view in the hospital room, staring at Dave, we no longer felt so lucky. We'd been owed one? Well, we'd gotten one. The big doozy I'd been bracing for—it was here.

I remember that during our first weeks at RIC, I was sitting with Dave in a speech therapy session when he was asked to name as many fruits and vegetables as he could in one minute. He could come up with three. He was asked to provide a woman's name that begins with each successive letter of the alphabet. He could not get past the letter "A." My name begins with the letter "A."

We made Dave a little calendar that we would look over, hour after hour, day after day. We cut out a Post-it that said "TODAY IS:" and we would slide that over the new square on the calendar at the start of each new day. Throughout the day, we would reference that calendar, reminding Dave where he was and why he was there. We would go over photos with him and review names. We would ask him trivia; he somehow always retained all the sports trivia in his head. Priorities, I guess.

We watched DVDs, too, specifically home videos that his brother and father had brought in. At one point, I asked Dave if he wanted me to bring in the DVD of our wedding. "No," he answered, quietly.

"Why not?" I asked, but I already knew. I offered him the answer: "Do you think it would make you sad to see it?"

He nodded his head, yes.

"OK. Then we will wait and watch that one together at home."

Dave fatigued easily and was usually ready for bed by seven. I would wait until he was asleep, sitting beside his bed, typing out my letter journal entry, and then drive home. Returning to our apartment at the end of each day was painful.

By day, I was the stalwart spouse, the hopeful wife who put on a happy face for the doctors and nurses and therapists, for my in-laws and the endless stream of family and friends who visited and, most important, for Dave. I was optimistic and strong and earned compliments like, "I can't believe how well you're holding up."

But at night, once I was alone and the armor was shed, I was sad. I was sad and lonely and so terribly frightened. Exhausted as I was, I had a hard time sleeping. I missed Dave's physical presence at home and in bed, yes, but more so I missed the part of him that was utterly absent, even when I sat beside him in his room at rehab; I missed the intangibles that made him Dave. I missed the life we had built together. Everything at home reminded me of how far removed our former life suddenly was, perhaps irretrievably so. The Blue Italian dishes we had received as wedding gifts and had eaten off of together countless times. Photos of us: on a boat ride during our honeymoon in Australia, on a ski trip to Vermont during Dave's medical school, in the basement of a college fraternity house dressed in tie-dyed aerobics outfits. Little handwritten notes that we had written each other that were tucked in random places around our apartment. The doctor's white coat hanging in the closet, on it clipped the hospital employee ID card in which Dave smiled, so handsome. So strong and healthy, Dr. David Levy.

One of the most painful things was Dave's Hawaii suitcase.

When I first brought it home, Penny sniffed it, tail wagging, presuming that this item that smelled so full of Dave was a precursor to the real thing returning. She ran around the apartment, seeking him out, but he did not appear.

I let the suitcase sit there, unopened, for several weeks. I did not want to look through it and think of the Tuesday afternoon when Dave had packed it. I did not want to see his familiar clothes, an iPod that he would have listened to while he worked out. Flip-flops he would have worn to the beach. His passport for our day trip from Seattle to Vancouver. The sunglasses we had picked out together before his laser eye surgery. Shirts of his that—yes, I did this, I'm embarrassed to admit it, but I did—still smelled like him. Artifacts of a trip never taken, a life now gone, snatched from us so suddenly.

I put it off as long as I could, but eventually I needed some of the items in that suitcase for Dave at rehab. I sat down on the floor with the dreaded thing. I girded myself to open it up and confront the items that had belonged to the old Dave, back when Dave would have known how to pack a suitcase. But when I went to unzip it, I discovered that it was locked. A four-digit passcode was required to open the lock.

Dave usually used the same four-digit passcode any time one was required. In fact, it had been one of the most interesting moments on our honeymoon, when he had let me in on his four-digit passcode while locking the safe in our hotel room in Port Douglas. *What about* my *four-digit passcode, the one I always like to use?* I'd thought. It dawned on me in that moment: I was married. Life would be different, being part of a duo, having to negotiate who got to choose the four-digit hotel safe passcode. I take thee, David, with your four-digit passcode, forsaking all others. . . . So this was marriage.

But to my surprise, Dave's suitcase was not opening with that now-familiar four-digit combination. Stumped, I sat back. Asking

Dave would have been impossible; he could not remember what a suitcase was, let alone that he had packed one for Hawaii, let alone what its security combination might be. I tried various configurations including birthdays and addresses and other significant dates. God, how I missed him, how I wished he could have been there to tell me the code. Or better yet, to unpack the suitcase himself. Or, even better still, to have unpacked the suitcase *after* getting to have that trip, that babymoon, in that other life that we had planned.

One night when I was feeling particularly desperate and maudlin, I considered calling Dave's cellphone. I knew it was turned off—it was sitting in our bedroom on our bedside table, off since that horrible June 9 flight—but that was precisely the idea. I would get his voicemail and I could listen to the sound of his voice, his *real* voice. Since waking up, Dave was speaking in this voice and this cadence that was just not him; his voicemail would give me ten seconds of that old Dave voice. But I realized that that was completely mawkish and would facilitate a spiral of self-pity that would probably result in me weeping in the fetal position. Not productive. So I forced myself not to call his cellphone.

The thing that nearly broke me was that, several weeks into RIC, I had to move apartments. Our lease was up, and the plan had always been to move a week after our babymoon, at the end of June; we just hadn't planned on the stroke. The logistics of any move are tough, but when you are spending twelve hours a day in the hospital and you are forbidden by your doctor from lifting heavy objects at six months pregnant, it becomes even more problematic. I did not know how I could possibly make it happen. Not to mention that packing would mean reckoning with item after item from Dave's and my former life, pouring saltwater into a fresh wound with each one.

All I can say is this: thank God for women. Women show up. And the women in my life showed up for me at that time, in every way. My friend Marya flew out to help me pack up our old place. Marya was exactly the right person to arrive in that moment because she, more so than any other friend, has known Dave since the earliest days of our courtship. She first introduced me to him, on that night when he asked me where I went to college at a Yale bar. She was in that same art history class. She witnessed me sliding in next to Dave to learn about Gothic cathedrals. She stood beside us at the altar when we got married. I could be entirely raw and vulnerable—broken—in front of her. And Marya missed Dave, too. Not just for me, but because of her own long friendship with him.

When I answered the door, I saw Marya and immediately collapsed into her outstretched arms. She held me and wept with me. This was no small mercy, to have someone simply allow me to cry. She did not look for a positive piece of loving wisdom. She did not try to cheer me up. She just held me and she let me cry, and she cried with me.

"I just miss him so much," I said, as we drove together one morning to see Dave in rehab. Tears in her eyes, she nodded. "I know you do," she said. "But he's still here," she offered. I knew her point was: *He's not dead.* It was true. He very well might have been dead. In spite of the hideousness of the current situation, there was still reason to give thanks.

"It's a cruel, sick joke," she agreed with me. "You couldn't have made it up: you were on your way to your babymoon and your husband almost dies from a stroke."

Marya was there with me that weekend, overseeing the logistics of our life going into boxes. Our friends Peter and Russell came over and spackled the walls, took the TV screens out of their mounts, helped with packing, canceled our cable subscription.

Also during that time, Marya walked Penny over to RIC, and Dave and I went down to the street so he could see our dog for the first time since the stroke. It was not the reunion I had hoped for—Dave did not recognize our dog, and, even more strangely, Penny did not recognize Dave. Ordinarily she would have been beside herself, pouncing on him, yelping, running circles around his legs in her excitement at such a long-overdue reunion (she had not seen him all month, since the afternoon we had left for Hawaii). But now, rather than euphoric, Penny was scared; she shied away from him and cowered behind my legs. Was Dave really so changed that he had become unrecognizable to our family pet?

"You probably just smell like the hospital; she can't find your familiar scent," I said, trying to hide how heartbreaking I found it. In reality, I wanted to cry. Dave and Penny had always been so bonded that at times we had joked that I was the third wheel. In that moment, I wanted nothing more than to be the third wheel in the midst of their happy reunion. I wanted them to know and love each other, just as they always had, instead of meeting as distant and distrustful strangers.

Looking on, watching this tepid reunion, was Marya. She, too, was unrecognizable to Dave, and that broke her heart, both as a friend to me but also as a friend to Dave of more than a decade. Marya—or as Dave had always called her, Mar Mar—kept it together on the surface; she forced a smile even as, inside, she wanted to cry.

Marya returned to the hospital the next day, without Penny, to visit Dave one more time. As she walked down the hallway, she felt nervous and sad, dreading another visit with this replacement-Dave, a stranger who did not know her, had no recollection of their eleven years of friendship and the easy, playful banter that they had always enjoyed.

As Marya rounded the corner and entered the hospital room,

our friend Russell, who was also visiting, turned to Dave. "Hey, hey, recognize who just walked in?" Russell asked.

Dave, with a mischievous smirk on his face, a faint twinkle in his eye, nodded.

"Oh, yeah?" Russell prodded. "Who is she?"

Dave shrugged, turning his glance sideways. "Some bitch named Marya."

It was only at that point that Marya finally burst into the tears she had been holding back for the past couple of days. "Dave," she said, beaming through her tears, "those are the most beautiful words I have ever heard come out of your mouth!"

We all laughed—relieved at Marya's unruffled reaction, startled by Dave's off-color remark. It is not uncommon for stroke patients to speak with socially unacceptable bluntness or vulgarity, but this particular moment was funny because it *was* vestigial of the teasing, playful sparring that Dave and his Mar Mar had always shared. He was trying to make a joke. In its own odd and embarrassing way, we took it as a good sign.

The day Marya left, the day of the actual move, my in-laws were covering the early part of the day with Dave at rehab so that I could oversee the movers as they transferred our life from the old place to the new one. But just as I arrived at our new, empty apartment to await the moving truck, our new building's manager told me that Dave needed to sign the lease before we could occupy the apartment. Dave had planned to go into the leasing office and sign when we returned from Hawaii—clearly that had never happened. I hurried up to the rehabilitation facility, tracked down the social worker a second before she had to leave for a meeting, begged her to write a note explaining the situation on the requisite official RIC letterhead, and hurried back downtown to offer the letter and plead with the leasing office. The building allowed us to proceed with the move, given the circumstances. We were back on.

Then I heard from the movers, telling me that there was some delay with the moving truck. They were running a couple of hours behind. This was not good. Since the elevator in the new building was only available to us for the next two hours, our window was tight. The new building rented out the elevator in specific two-hour time blocks, and thus they could only honor the couple of hours for which I'd reserved it—after that, someone else had use of the elevator for *their* move. What the heck was I going to do with a moving truck full of boxes if I could not get it all from the truck into the new apartment? And where would I sleep? I pleaded with the movers to get there as fast as was humanly possible, in order to try to make our move-in window.

As I awaited the moving truck, nervously watching the clock tick forward, I decided to walk around the new neighborhood. It was the middle of the day, and I was starving. I scoped out the unfamiliar terrain. There was a sushi place, but I was not allowed to eat raw fish. There was a deli, but they only had cold sandwich meats—I was not supposed to eat those, either. "Do you have anything other than cold cuts?" I asked. "Cheese," they countered. So I ordered my cheese sandwich and headed back to the apartment. As I was crossing the street, the skies opened up. I had not known it was going to rain, and, besides, all my umbrellas were in a box somewhere, hopefully on their way to me in a moving truck. The rain pounded me, and within minutes I was soaked. I had no change of clothes, or dry shoes—those were packed. I felt like raising my cheese-sandwich-laden fist to the heavens and shouting out the question foremost on my mind: "Why, God? Why? What more do you plan to throw at me?"

I returned to my apartment with my soggy sandwich. As I stood there in the bare surroundings, standing at the kitchen counter, shivering in the air-conditioning because my clothes were doused, my dad called to see how the move was going. I could barely answer, "Not good," before bursting into tears. It was interesting, being able to reflect on the day I was having and to think, *This just might be one of the worst days of my entire life.*

The movers arrived, finally, and we raced to unload everything in time. I disregarded the fact that I was not supposed to lift heavy things—we needed all hands on deck. At one point, as we were frantically hauling boxes into the apartment, one of the movers looked at me with a concerned expression and asked if I was going to go into labor early because of all the stress, and I just sat down on top of a cardboard box, unsure how to answer the question. I forced myself to do some deep breathing. My swollen, wet feet hurt; my lower back ached. I was freezing—my clothes and hair and skin still damp from the downpour, my body shivering from the stress and the chilly blasts of sterile air being blown by the air conditioner.

Once the movers left, I looked around: this new apartment smelled like cardboard and paint and wet carpet. The rooms were a mess of boxes and furniture too heavy for me to arrange. This place, this apartment that Dave and I had been so thrilled to find, so excited to begin our new chapter in ("This will be the baby's room!" "This will be the guest room so Mom can come and help with the baby!"), felt nothing like home; it was unfamiliar and bare and all wrong. "It's good that you are moving now; it'll be a fresh start," my parents had reasoned. But the start of what? And fresh, well, the only thing that felt fresh in that moment was my pain and my loneliness and my fear. "Raw" might have been the more appropriate word.

I could not even begin to think about unpacking, about setting up a home; I had to get to rehab and to Dave. I had explained to him the night before that I would be late the following day because I had to oversee the movers in the morning, but there was no way he would have remembered. Was he sad at rehab, wondering where I was? Was he scared? The thought broke my heart.

❖ ❖ ❖

Again, thank God for girlfriends. My friends Margaret and Charlotte flew out to help unpack and settle me in. Two more of the
world's all-time great people, Margaret and Charlotte are my old-
est friends. I have known Margaret since we were toddlers, and
Charlotte was my ever-present best friend from middle school
onward. While there with me, Margaret built bookshelves and
unpacked clothes and gave me prenatal yoga classes and prayed
beside me in bed. Charlotte, only one month less pregnant than I
was at the time, unpacked box after box and hung photos on the
walls and arranged our dishes and told me optimistic stories and
got her husband to do the heavy lifting for us.

These special, selfless friends gave me a home; they gave me a
physical space in which to feel settled in the midst of the most
unsettling experience of my entire life. They allowed me to spend
all day with Dave at rehab and not be distracted with the move.
On countless trips to Target, they stocked me with toilet paper
and groceries and lightbulbs and coat hangers. In fact, they went
to Target so many times that the employees there got to know
them, even lending them a Target cart to shuttle their goods back
to my place. One of my favorite stories from their Target trips was
when a woman in the checkout line took a look at their haul and
asked the natural question: "Did you ladies just move in?"

Not wanting to get into the whole complicated explanation,
Charlotte and Margaret just smiled and nodded, yes, they were
moving in. It was true—they were moving *me* in.

"Where are you from?" this fellow customer asked.

Again, Charlotte and Margaret went with the simple, easy answer. "We're from New York." Again, it *was* true.

The woman grinned, then glanced at Charlotte's baby bump.
"Your first baby?"

Charlotte nodded.

"How nice!" she said, a big smile on her face as she looked from Charlotte to Margaret. "Well, welcome to the neighborhood." It was then that Charlotte and Margaret realized that this woman presumed them to be a couple, moving in and preparing for their first baby. We had a good laugh that night over takeout on the roof of my new building.

I could not believe how much these girls, and so many others, were willing to do for Dave and me. My brother's wife, Emled, called her mother in from out of town to help my brother watch their two little ones so that she could fly out and keep me company for a week, showing me how to set up baby gear and unpacking our final boxes. My sister, Emily, at home awaiting a new baby, checked in constantly. My sister-in-law Marie brought me lunch at RIC. Friends sent food and baby gifts and flowers and so much love. One friend sent me a gift certificate for a prenatal massage and a note reminding me to take care of myself.

I was suddenly in the position where I had to take; I had to draw on my tribe for support and strength. I did not feel comfortable with that; it felt one-sided. I felt—no, I *worried*—that I was putting people out, inconveniencing them. I referred to myself as "the high-needs friend," and I hated that. I bristled at the idea of *needing* that much. When I confessed this fear to Margaret, she looked me in the eyes and said, "Alli, we *want* to do this for you. Don't you see? It gives us joy to feel that we can carry just a little bit of your burden for you. We are God's hands for you."

I needed them, and I accepted that. It was the season of life that I was in, and I was lucky that all of these people showed up for me and for Dave in the ways they did. All I could do was hope that the season would pass, that at some point I would get back to the place where I would feel strong and where life would feel stable enough that I could return the love.

Chapter 22

DAVE'S REHAB FLOOR AT RIC AFFORDED GLORIOUS PANORAMIC views of Lake Michigan, and on the Fourth of July, we looked out over an expanse of shimmering blue water dotted with boats. Music traveled up to us on the warm air and rattled our windows. The beach was packed, and our view was filled with people swimming, laughing, reveling.

That week was to have been the first week of Dave's fourth year of residency.

Dave's parents drove down the morning of the Fourth of July, his mother bringing us sweets and baked goods, before heading back north to join the rest of the family for a parade. How I envied them all the ability to do something as ordinary and carefree as go to a parade. There is just something about holidays and happy times that makes it so much harder when you yourself are in pain. It is hard to feel deeply unhappy on any day—but all the more so when you are confronted, like on a holiday, with so many other people who just look and seem so darn *happy*.

Our friends Lizzie and Kevin came to RIC that afternoon, and the four of us walked outside to the lake. It was Dave's first outing far from the RIC campus without medical supervision, and he was not himself—unsteady on his feet and not entirely coherent when he spoke—so we joked that everyone would assume he was just another reveler who had perhaps enjoyed too many adult beverages.

We were one month out from the stroke, and I was still running on adrenaline and positivity. But I could not ignore the fear and confusion and discomfort I saw on the faces of some of the friends who visited. I knew some people had to be thinking, *Thank God this didn't happen to me.* It was only natural. One particular remark that stung was when the wife of a visitor told me she had "hugged her husband extra close in bed the night before, thinking about how it could have been him." I knew people had to be thinking that, of course. Candidly, I would have had the same thought had the places been reversed, but she did not win any awards for empathy by saying it aloud.

In an email to Dave's friends updating them on the move to RIC and letting them know about the policies for visitors, Andy laid out some basic facts to prepare people for what to expect. He asked people to project positivity during their visits; to talk to Dave and ask him questions and try to trigger fond memories and associations. Andy wrote, **"I know it's sad to see a guy wearing Yale Lacrosse shorts who can't cut his own food."** Yes, it was, I realized, when I saw it spelled out so plainly in writing.

May we always remember how lucky we are.

After long days in the hospital, I would return home to our empty apartment and I would see that photo of the four-leaf clovers and I would want to tear it off the wall and hurl it across the room. What had I been thinking, writing such a thing? Had I really needed to tempt the fates like that? Had I needed to revel in my good luck, gloating before the gods, daring them to rob me of my fortune?

Sometimes I would stare at my iPhone calendar and lust after the life of June 8. I'd relive the moments and days that predated the stroke, all of them now washed in a blissful, halcyon glow of bygone innocence and ease. I would rewatch the iPhone video from the day, just a week before the stroke, when we found out we were having a girl—our shocked, delighted faces, our long hug. I would wallow in a temporary amnesia that pretended that life was as it had once been, back when the biggest problem was a parking ticket or a tight work deadline. I would barter in my head, negotiating with God: "If only you will give me Dave back, I promise I will . . ."

May we always remember.

Remember? Dave could not even remember what city we lived in. He could not remember our anniversary. He could not remember the name of our beloved pet dog.

Fatigue, too, was a constant combatant. Dave would nap between most therapy sessions, on top of thirteen hours of sleep each night. At bedtime I would cuddle him—full light outside the window, these being the longest days of the year—in the narrow hospital bed until he fell asleep. As he drifted off, I would pray for healing. I would pray that the Holy Spirit would work miracles in that room and inside his head.

In our old life, the life before his stroke, our bedtime ritual had been very different. I was always the one who took longer to get ready—all Dave had to do was brush his teeth, whereas I would brush my teeth and take out my contact lenses and wash my face and apply a whole lineup of toners and lotions. Dave would lie in bed, battling sleep. "Hurry up, I'm falling asleep!"

I'd hurry through the rest of my routine and then hop into bed beside him and Penny (yes, we let our dog sleep with us). Dave would wrap his arms around us, a big sandwich, and he would say, sighing: "This is my idea of heaven."

One night at RIC when I got in bed with him to snuggle before sleep, I told him about that. "You'd always say: 'This is my idea of heaven.' Do you remember that?"

He shook his head. Marya, visiting, had witnessed our night-time hospital ritual, and so, several weeks later, a pillow showed up with Penny's face on it. She wanted the three of us to be able to continue our bedtime ritual. So each night we would snuggle, the two of us and my big belly and the Penny pillow, and I would say, "This is my idea of heaven." I would fight back the tears as I hoped that one day Dave would remember that ritual from our old life. That one day we would return to the place where he would hurry me through my nighttime face-washing and I could hop into bed and he could say: This is my idea of heaven.

The days were long and full of rehab, and I continued to add to my DearDave Word document each night. I would write as the sun dipped through the window over Lake Michigan. I would look from Dave's sleeping figure around the darkening room. Just beside the bed, the digital picture frame our friend Russell had sent would be rotating through photos, the scenes of our former life on an endless loop. Dave, suntanned and relaxed with our friends in Lake George. Dave and me, jubilant, running out of the church on our wedding day as flower petals rain down. Dave, proud, standing next to his father at his medical school gradua-tion. Dave playing lacrosse in college. Each photo was a fresh punch in the gut. The shards of a life that had once belonged to two very different people.

Dear Dave,

Holding you tonight, watching you drift off to sleep, I wept silently, not wanting to wake you up. This digital picture frame in your hospital room reminds me of so many joyful memories, so many memories that, now, hurt to look at. Will you ever come back to me in the same smiling, strong, glorious form as the one in the pictures I now see? God, I miss you.

There's a phrase I like, one that I have told myself often during hard times. *It's always darkest before the dawn.* I do not know whether that was necessarily the darkest moment; there would be no point in trying to identify that. It was a dark moment, but it is certainly true that a major spear of light followed shortly after.

Chapter 23

New York
November 2011

DAVE AND I WERE MARRIED EXACTLY TWO MONTHS BEFORE I realized that life had completely changed.

Dave had just begun his fourth and final year of medical school, and we were now looking ahead to the next step in his training. Residency would be five years, and he would be training in orthopedic surgery. Dave cast a wide net, applying to programs all over the country.

His first interview was at Duke, a place where he had nearly gone for undergraduate, the place where his parents had met and courted and spent the early years of their marriage. Dave loved Duke, and he called me from his residency interview elated, telling me: "Alli, you'd love it here. Forget our one-bedroom apartment, we could have a *house* for what we pay in rent." Next was UCLA, and I got the phone call: "You'd love it out here. It's seventy degrees in the middle of winter. You'd be far from your family, but think how often they'd want to visit!" He loved most of the places he saw. I went on this roller coaster beside him, Googling apartment rentals in each subsequent city or town, wrapping my head around each possible plunge that we might take together.

Ultimately, though, it came down to two places: Columbia in New York City and Rush in Chicago. Dave, being from Chicago, was predisposed to like the programs there, but he especially loved the program at Rush University Medical Center, which he believed could not be more perfectly suited to him. He had also enjoyed his time at Columbia and had a close relationship with several of the attending orthopedic surgeons and therefore gave serious consideration to continuing there.

Programs aside, in our perfect worlds, Dave wanted to be in Chicago and I wanted to be in New York. I had grown up in New York. Heck, not only had I grown up in New York, I had grown up in "I Love New York" commercials. My family and most of my closest friends were there. I wanted to be a writer, and much of the publishing world and media were headquartered in New York City. But as passionate as I felt about New York, as rooted as I felt there, that was exactly how Dave felt about his hometown near Chicago. So, what were we to do?

This was, without a doubt, the single greatest challenge our relationship had faced to that point. We both loved our families and friends and were both eager to work in the city where we felt most rooted—so who got to win this one?

Dave got the message through the orthopedic grapevine that if he *really* liked a program much more than all the others, if there was one program that he knew he wanted to rank at the top of his list, it would help significantly to let that program know how serious he was about going there. "Alli, I think I should tell Rush that they are my first choice."

He told me this one night over the phone as I was wrapping up work and preparing to head to dinner with some girlfriends. I paused, irritated. Dave had not even completed all of his New York interviews yet. There was a big one coming up at a really competitive New York program; couldn't he at least try to keep an open mind and not shut the door on the idea of New York until he had at least seen all of the options? What if he fell in love with a New York program?

The night before, I had heard Dave in the other room on the phone with his dad, practicing for an upcoming interview. "My greatest achievement? Easy. My greatest achievement is, without a doubt, marrying my wife," Dave had said. Now I thought: *Well, excuse me, if I'm really your greatest achievement, then can't you please think about my perspective here?*

But he was running out of time to let Rush know—he'd already interviewed there and he had heard through the rumor mill that Rush would be ranking their applicants in the next day or so. If he wanted to rank in their top five and thus stand his best chance of getting into his dream program, it made sense for him to at least let them know how much he loved it there. I dug in. I withheld my blessing for such a conversation. It all struck me as premature and unfairly rushed; I felt it was only fair that he finish his interviews and give the New York programs a shot before committing us to a move I was not crazy about, one that I worried could pull me away from my own career opportunities in New York.

We took a few hours apart, both of us tense and frustrated that the other one seemed to be calling the shots over our respective futures. Dave called Louisa and spoke with her. Louisa then called me. It is a testament to my mother-in-law and the remarkable woman she is that she listened to each of us with complete fairness and open-minded understanding. She helped us each to see the other's perspective, and she urged us to communicate in a respectful and considerate manner.

In the end, I told Dave to have the conversation he had been wanting to have—to let Rush know they were at the top of his list. He answered by telling me that he had decided not to do it, to keep his mind open until he was done with all of his New York interviews. It was like our own version of the O. Henry story. We would hold off on making our rank list . . . for now. But the big unanswered question loomed, and we still had not sorted out how we would answer it.

Then something happened that was very hard, and that, in turn, made our decision very easy. If the question of Chicago versus New York was some choppy water rocking our marital boat, we soon forgot about that choppy water when we realized that we were smack dab in the middle of a hurricane.

I remember the phone call. It was early February, just a few days before Dave's birthday and Valentine's Day and the day Dave had to submit his final rank list for residency.

It was the middle of the day, and I was at work at my father's consulting group in Midtown Manhattan, where I did work researching and writing. For the past few months, my mother-in-law had been feeling pain in her back. In recent weeks it had gotten worse, and physical therapy was not helping. Her voice was shaky on the phone, entirely unlike her usually chipper tone. "It's the Big C," Louisa told me. Cancer. My mother-in-law had been diagnosed with multiple myeloma, a rare cancer of the blood. They say that "there is cancer, and then there is CANCER." Well, this was CANCER. No cure exists as of yet for multiple myeloma, and we were told that the life expectancy was just a couple of years.

I called Dave immediately. He was up on the Columbia campus in Washington Heights, and he broke down, sobbing into the phone. He had spoken with his parents right before I had. He adored his mother—everyone who knew her adored Louisa, and

Dave was her baby. He was a mess. "I can't be away from her as she's going through this, Alli. We've got to be in Chicago. I need to be near her."

I could feel the anguish in his voice—fear, helplessness, the overpowering desire to be near his mother during the coming months of uncertainty and hardship and physical pain. "Of course you do," I said.

We put Rush University number one and University of Chicago number two, to ensure that we would end up near Dave's family. In the end, fighting over which city to live in felt like a luxury compared to the news that a loved one might not live.

Chapter 24

Dear Dave,

You are working so hard. I am so proud of you. Watching you on the treadmill, hooked up to a harness and practicing hand-eye coordination exercises with balls and balloons, singing at the top of your lungs to Billy Joel, I've never been more in awe of you or more in love with you.

Today while you had your hour-long occupational therapy session I went for a walk along Lake Michigan. I'm starting to feel things again, small things, like appreciation for sunshine. I'm smiling back at people who comment on my baby bump. I'm coming back to life along with you.

Dear Dave,

Today was a day of ups and downs. In your psychology consult, you had a frank conversation with Dr. Pratt about what happened to you, and it seemed like one of the first times that it really sank in. You got really sad. Your entire demeanor seemed *to sag. You told us that you felt sad, that you felt like you weren't your old self, that you didn't understand why this stroke had happened to you. It took all I had not to burst into tears right there; I wanted to be strong for you. I told you that I felt sad, too. That I didn't understand it, either. But that I know you will beat this. That I do not want to call anything a "silver lining" in this shitty situation, but that I know, somehow, somewhere down the road, we will find positives out of this hell. That it has been the worst three weeks of your life, and that fighting your way back after this stroke will be the hardest challenge you will ever face, but that there is no doubt in my mind that you will win this fight. That we will win this fight together. And that, in the end, you will not only be 100 percent of yourself, but that you will be 110 percent of yourself. That, after surviving this hell, you will come out of it with a greater appreciation for life and all of its beauty. Hey, you are ALIVE. Let's start with that: you are still here with us. I have never been more grateful for anything in my life. You are here and you will get better and at the end of this, I believe you will have an entirely new outlook on life. You will be a better man and an even better husband and brother and son and friend. An even better doctor. An even better father. A kinder, gentler, more appreciative man.*

Fortunately, we followed that psych talk with physical therapy, which you always love. We hooked you up to the anti-gravity machine, which was pretty cool, and you ran with 50 percent of your body weight. You enjoyed that, though you did comment (ALOUD!) that it "made your balls feel weird." The PT really liked that one. Yikes. Following your PT session you had a steady stream of visitors. You had a childhood friend from Lake Forest, Teddy; you had a college friend, Peter; and you had a residency friend, Will. Three friends from three different phases of your life all in one room because they love you so much. You laughed big time. Your mood totally lifted as you recalled childhood memories and listened to the latest residency gossip.

We ended the day on a high note. In bed, I repeated our daily mantra: "Every day, in every way, I'm getting better and better." I asked you if you truly believed that and you told me you did. I couldn't stop hugging you. I'm just so happy to have you here. You are so beautiful to me. Watching you sleep, your face innocent, your body tucked up snugly under the white blankets, you look so peaceful. I hope you are dreaming wonderful dreams. I have always loved to watch you sleep (sorry if that sounds creepy)—I have. You just look so . . . at rest. But now even more so. OK, you have an early morning tomorrow with the breakfast group, and I need to get home to walk our sweet pup. I love you. Sleep tight and dream happy dreams, my love. May this sleep tonight be restorative and healing and peaceful, and may God be working miracles in your brain and your body. I love you.

Dear Dave,

You were wiped at the end of today, after two outdoor excursions and a kick-butt PT session, so now you are in bed. We spoke about the exciting few days we have coming up, and you asked if you could sleep at home on Sunday when you have your day off. My heart aches, because God, how I wish you could sleep at home. A little over two weeks left of this—you know that I am counting down the mornings, days, and nights. In the meantime, I love you so much and there is nowhere else I would rather be than here in this room with you.

Dear Dave,

Today was a good day. I picked you up at ten A.M. with Peter and Jackie. We took you to your favorite restaurant for Sunday brunch. *You were so excited to be out in the world and at your favorite spot that you were a bit goofy and a bit impulsive with your language, but that's OK. You ordered your go-to smoothie and ate an omelet and then we walked the short distance to our new place.*

I loved showing you around our new place, loved watching you see all of your familiar items, beloved photos, worn-in furniture. But the best was just how happy you and Penny were to be reunited. She jumped on you so excitedly that you have scratches on your arms now to show for it. She cried and whimpered and licked and showed you how much she'd been missing you. Together, we walked her to her new dog park and you cleaned up her poop. Then, we came back, and this next part was quite possibly my favorite part of the entire day: we did nothing. We did absolutely nothing, but we did it together, and we did it at home. We snuggled on the couch and talked about our new apartment. We both dozed off and took naps (all three of us, if you count Penny).

We woke up just in time for our visitors. Your friend Steffen came and your parents came and Erin and Annabel and Will, and Mike and Marie and Cooper. It was happy chaos in our apartment, with you loving your screaming niece and nephews. We walked around the new building and checked out the rooftop lounge and sundeck. We walked with the kids to the dog park and played outside a bit. Annabel kept trying to put the pebbles from the dog park into her mouth. Then we came inside and ordered Lou Malnati's pizza. It was such a good day. Such a good day that I didn't know how I would survive the fact that it was over.

When it was time to come back to RIC, we were both incredibly sad and tearful—we snuggled the entire car ride back as your parents drove us. I just keep trying to remind us both that it's only two weeks until you are out for good. How amazing will that feel, to be together every day? We will never take it for granted again.

Dear Dave,

The beginning of another week. Our second to last week. We just need to get through this. You are starting to become more aware, which is an awesome thing. But, as you become more aware, you are starting to ask questions. You are starting to realize the enormity of what happened to you, and that brings with it a heavy medley of emotions.

Dear Dave,

It sounds so cliché, but you really are getting better and better each day, and it is so exciting to see.

You and your dad went through all of the characters in The Lord of the Rings *today.*

Dear Dave,

Today was another day forward. John L was here—he flew in for the day just to visit you. You were loaded up because tomorrow is a day off, so today you had two physical therapies and an occupational therapy session. No nap. We walked outside—you took John to the beach and we sat in the park.

By this evening you were completely wiped. As you were settling into bed, you asked me what happened and I went through the whole thing with you and there was an awareness and a comprehension that I haven't seen yet.

At first you felt really good and optimistic as I laid out all of the reasons why you should feel hopeful and proud and encouraged. You liked my line that you are "my superhero."

You shut your eyes.

And then you opened them. And you turned to me. And your face was so strained and tense that I literally thought you were playing with me, like, teasing me. You've been in a very teasing and playful humor all day. So I asked: "Are you joking, trying to freak me out right now?" I thought you were kidding around, it was such an extreme look, and one I have never seen before. But you shook your head, no, you weren't doing this in jest. So I got up and came to your bed and asked what was wrong and your answer was: "I'm scared."

So we talked about your situation again and I laid out just how many people are here for you and advocating for you and with you. That you will not ever be alone on this journey. That I am here beside you at every step of the way, as is your entire family and all of your friends.

But you told me that you are scared because on Monday you are to go to the John Hancock building with your speech therapy group. You are scared to be in that tall building. You're scared you might get left up there or you might fall off the building. So I asked you if it would make you feel better if I joined you and you said yes, so I will come to the John Hancock building with you on Monday.

And then I told you a story. I told you that every night before I leave your hospital room, I pray over your sleeping figure. I pray for Jesus to hold you in the palm of his hand so that you would have rest and peace and hope and comfort and healing. I pray that the Holy Spirit would be working in this room and in your brain and in your body and in the capable hands and minds of your incredible medical team. And I pray that angels would be surrounding your bed all through the night. I told you that on the flight from Fargo to Chicago, we flew at the same time but I was on a commercial flight and you were on a medical plane. I prayed the whole flight that there would be angels surrounding your plane and inside your plane, overwhelming you with grace and safety and peace and comfort. And I know there were—because my plane went through terrible turbulence on that flight; yours went through none at all. I told you that I believed that that was because the angels were guiding your plane and making your path smooth, as they will continue to do. We must continue to have faith.

You liked that. You also said: "Gosh, I've been through a lot."

That's the understatement of the year, to be sure. But the fact that you made such a statement is promising to me. It shows me that you are processing and reflecting and understanding and reacting. You have been through a lot, and you realize it.

Chapter 25

"WHAT'S THE NAME OF MY DOG?"

"Wanda!" Dave exclaimed, smiling as he said it.

"Wanda the . . . ?"

"Wanda the Wonder-dog!"

That became the daily greeting between Dave and his rehabilitation physician, as Dr. Richard Harvey would stroll into our room, flanked by residents and trainees, early each morning on his daily rounds.

Dr. Harvey was another one of the colorful and kind characters who entered our lives in the months of the stroke and recovery and quickly became a member of our team. The head of physical medicine and rehabilitation at RIC, Dr. Harvey was a tall, lanky man with big glasses and a big smile, a stethoscope draped around his neck. He loved yoga and mindfulness, he believed in the importance of staying optimistic, and he always wore his pants just a tad short, revealing a colorful sampling of his quirky sock collection.

Having learned that Dave was a dog lover, Dr. Harvey began to use questions about his own dog as one of his daily orienting tests for memory. At first, Dave could not remember that Dr. Harvey had a dog. Then, after a few days of repetition, Dave could remember the dog but not the name. "I want you to remember, Dave: my dog's name is Wanda. OK? Wanda the Wonder-dog." Dr. Harvey pulled out his phone and scrolled through a series of pictures of Wanda: frolicking near the lake in Michigan, sunning herself in the grass, leaping to catch a ball. "Tomorrow I'm going to ask you again, OK? Remember Wanda. It will be part of your daily orienting test to see how your memory is doing."

"All right," Dave agreed. Would he be able to remember? I wondered. Physically, Dave was getting stronger each day. His balance was improving, he could climb a few stairs, and we would soon be able to take him outside for longer walks. But his memory improvement was lagging. Several times throughout the day, in addition to asking Dave about the date and location, I now started asking him: "What's the name of Dr. Harvey's dog?"

I tried to be there for these morning visits between Dave and Dr. Harvey. For starters, I liked Dr. Harvey. His daily positivity and humor were refreshing, and it was my chance to confer, my time to ask questions or relay questions from Dave's other family members.

One morning in midsummer I hurried down the hall to make it in time for the early rounds. My routine was to wake up, walk the dog, eat a quick breakfast, and get into RIC. That day, however, when I strolled into Dave's room, it was empty. I guessed that I had missed Dr. Harvey. Knowing that Dave could be in only one of three places—physical therapy, occupational therapy, or speech therapy—I sought him out on the floor. He was not in the rooms where speech therapy and OT were held, so I made my way down the hall to the gym for PT. As I neared, I could hear music and laughter.

Like all inpatients, Dave was not allowed to use the treadmill without being hooked up to straps that hung from the ceiling, in case he lost his balance and fell. Frankly, it was sort of sad to see: my strong husband, an athlete who had won every physical accolade the college athletics department had offered, now so unsteady that he could not so much as walk on a treadmill without what looked like a horse harness. And yet, that day, I did not notice that. That day, I noticed that when I walked into the gym, Dave was walking sideways on the treadmill. To be more precise, Dave was dancing, doing the grapevine, injecting a fair amount of rhythm and sass into his steps as he kept time to the song playing on the gym loudspeakers. I still remember the song, by a group called Walk the Moon. It's a fun, upbeat melody, the type of song that, in another life, Dave and I would have loved dancing to at a wedding.

> *I said you're holding back*
> *She said shut up and dance with me!*

I stopped in my tracks and watched. There Dave was, dancing on the treadmill while throwing a ball with one therapist and answering another therapist's trivia questions. My mouth fell open. I looked at the nearest physical therapist, and she nodded at me as if to say, *I know, right?* What she said aloud was: "He's cracking us all up with his moves!"

Dave and I love to dance. We are both terrible dancers—my moves are just slightly better than Elaine's on *Seinfeld,* on a good day—but we love to dance. We fell in love dancing. Our courtship in college played out largely to dancing, primarily at a seedy New Haven bar called Toad's Place, where one can get beer for a penny and dance (when one's shoes aren't sticking to the floor) to a predictable playlist of Bon Jovi and Journey and Michael Jackson. Here Dave was, dancing his heart out as if he were back at Toad's—having a blast doing it and making us all laugh as we looked on.

Dear Dave,

You kissed my belly and said, "Good night, Lilly," before going to sleep tonight. You kicked butt in PT—you walked sideways on the treadmill while throwing a ball and answering questions.

I'll be going home to our new apartment and it will be empty. My goodness, I miss you.

All of the memories that were supposed to be ours, would have been ours in an alternate life, a life when you had not suffered an inexplicable stroke at age thirty. It feels so cruel. So today when I see you I cling to you and tell you how much I love you, and I can't stop thinking Thank God you are still here with me. *I'm watching you fight sleep, your eyes slowly getting heavier, and all I can think about is that I just love you so much.*

There were ups and downs every single day. My sister gave birth to her second child, a healthy baby boy, that July, and Dave and I were able to FaceTime her just a few moments after her delivery to "meet" our little nephew.

The next day was clear and sunny, so Dave and I decided to take a walk to the nearby beach during one of his breaks in therapy. As we crossed Lake Shore Drive, we passed a police car. Dave turned to me and said: "I feel like screaming at this cop. Can I yell at him?"

"No! You can't scream at him," I whispered sternly, and hurried Dave across the street and away from the police car.

As he was recovering, glimmers of Dave's personality were beginning to emerge, but a lot of the time he basically seemed like an intoxicated or juvenile caricature of his former self. It was pretty common for him to burst into outrageous and offensive epithets directed at strangers.

"Hey, move aside, slowpokes!" Now, as we walked the crowded footpath along Lake Michigan, just a few blocks from RIC, Dave shouted at a swimsuit-clad woman and her muscular companion. The woman looked at us, shocked. The guy beside her looked like he was ready to put his fists up. "Sorry!" I grimaced and quickly steered Dave away from the couple, wondering if perhaps we needed to end our outing before Dave got himself a black eye.

When Dave would yell these things at passersby, he did not mean to be combative or rude. In fact, he did not even know that he had done anything wrong—the drive center of his brain, the part that regulated impulse control, had been seriously damaged in the stroke, so he was completely uninhibited and often displayed questionable (to put it generously) judgment. He thought of these random outbursts as nothing more than hilarious jokes; the recipients of these "jokes" obviously saw things quite differently, and so taking Dave out in public was becoming increasingly challenging.

I pulled one of Dave's therapists aside to discuss this troubling new trend later that day, after he had tried to yell at the police officer. "I love to get outside with Dave when he has breaks in his therapy. It's good stimulation and good exercise to walk along the lake, and I think it's got to be good for his mood, but it's mortifying when he yells, even curses, at complete strangers. Today he almost yelled at a cop."

His speech therapist, Renee, nodded as she listened, and then offered me her thoughtful reply. "OK, so, immediately after the stroke, we struggled to get Dave to answer questions, much less initiate any communication on his own. Now he is initiating communication, but obviously not in the way we would like. This is pretty normal as his initiation comes back online. We will work on getting him to scale it back and focus on initiating and communicating in a way that is socially appropriate." Whatever I did, Renee warned me, we were *not* to laugh. I sent an email that night to his guy friends: **"Do NOT laugh at Dave's verbal outbursts. We should not be encouraging this."**

Other times Dave's demeanor was like that of a sweet, helpless child. This was most evident in the way he spoke. When not cursing like a sailor at random passersby, Dave was using a baby voice in pretty much every conversation. It was a voice I knew well— it's the voice he uses to speak affectionately to me and to our dog and to his mother. That was fine, but it was not particularly appropriate that Dave was cooing and crooning to his doctors and colleagues and therapists.

We had some fun as we tried to remind Dave to turn off that baby voice. "Dave, use your grown-up voice," Renee would urge him.

"Hello! How are you?" Dave would respond, speaking in a booming baritone, a playfully deep voice that sounded remarkably similar to Will Ferrell's imitation of Robert Goulet.

"That's your Newscaster Dave voice," Renee responded, smiling. "It's better. But now try to just sound like normal, grown-up Dave, not Baby Dave or Newscaster Dave."

"Hello," Dave would respond, his voice somewhere in the middle of his baby talk and his Robert Goulet.

In spite of my initial concern over depression, Dave was in remarkably good spirits, and he was improving. There were moments of celebrating, and there were plenty of moments when we genuinely laughed. Our room, with Dave as the merry center of a steady stream of friends and visitors, often had the feel of a lively cocktail party, minus the alcohol. One of his physical medicine doctors at RIC told us that visiting Dave was the highlight of her day because he was friendly, optimistic, and funny. But mostly because his improvements were so clear and noticeable.

My evening letter to Dave one night said:

Dear Dave,

You see, in many ways (most ways), these have been the worst weeks of my life. And they've been even worse for you. But, in some inexplicable way, they have been the most meaningful weeks of our life together. You and I are living out our marital vows every single day. That whole "for better or for worse, in sickness and in health" thing is playing out for us, hour by hour, day by day.

In so many ways, we have never been more connected. You see, you are a medical resident, and for as long as we have been married, we've never had enough time together. The demands of your work schedule always took you out of the home more than we wanted, always required sacrifices to be made. Now we spend twelve hours together a day, every single day. We talk about everything. We eat every meal together. We are so close that I know when the last time was that you peed. We are so close that when I look down at my phone for thirty seconds and look back at you, you are staring at me and ask me, "How are you?" You are sweet and affectionate. You seek out my hand when we walk. You want my company. I guess we are finally getting the time together that we wanted. I'm just so sorry that it had to be under these circumstances.

We are in this together, more than we have ever been in anything together. We are a team, and, together, we are fighting every single day. You are not alone in this. You and I are fighting together—we are fighting for our future. We are fighting for our life together. We are fighting to regain the beautiful memories of the past. We are fighting to restore the freedom that we always took for granted in the present. And we are fighting to make the dreams of our future possible. We are fighting for our little girl. We are fighting for this unborn daughter and the future babies we've always wanted to have. We will do this. Together.

After several weeks of inpatient therapy at RIC, Dave's entire re-habilitation team convened to discuss the situation and present us with their prognosis. At RIC they call it the Family Huddle. The morning of our Huddle I was petrified. What sort of a life would they predict for Dave, and therefore my family and me? How would I accept this new life, whatever they expected it to look like?

We assembled in a conference room. My mother-in-law, who had recently fallen on the stairs at home and broken her tailbone (Yes, actually. Was fate playing some sort of sick joke on our family?), could not sit down, so I remember her standing beside the table, hovering, while the rest of us sat there, tense and stone-faced.

The medical team began by presenting the assessment of Dave's cognitive therapists. They ran a test on Dave every morning called the Galveston Orientation and Amnesia Test (GOAT), a series of very basic questions that demonstrate how aware a person is of his or her surroundings. What is your name? What city are you in? When is your birthday? And so on.

A high-functioning adult scores somewhere between 80 and 100 on the GOAT. A person in a state of amnesia scores below a 75. To be considered out of amnesia, one had to score a 76 or higher for three consecutive days on the GOAT.

When Dave arrived at RIC, the rehab team told us, he had scored an 8 out of 100. They told us about his difficulty with short-term memory. His executive-functioning capacity was wiped out. This affected everything from his ability to initiate actions (I should do something about these smelly armpits by showering; I should eat the food on this plate in front of me; I should take this empty plate and put it in the dishwasher) to planning complex sequencing (first I'll wake up, then I'll get out of bed, then I'll go to the bathroom, then I'll get dressed). Executive functioning is what allows an adult to manage his or her own life, to accomplish the tasks of daily living as an autonomous and productive individual, what allows us to be the "executive," or the boss, of our lives. It's stuff that we do every single day, without even thinking about it.

Dave could not be expected to handle any of that on his own—the simplest activities of daily life required constant prompting and reminders. For example, he had to be told to put his sneakers on; then he had to be told to tie those sneakers; then he had to be told to stand up from the bed and go to whatever appointment he had to go to.

Additionally, since the stroke had targeted his thalamus, the portion of the brain that regulates the body's sleep and wakefulness, Dave's brain was telling him at all times that he was incredibly tired. This was why he needed so much sleep, both at night and with multiple daytime naps.

And yet, as we sat around the table that day at the Family Huddle, the medical team told us that their goal and their expectation was that Dave would make a full recovery. Factors such as his youth, his therapy plan, and his "pre-morbid condition"—that is, the state of Dave's functionality prior to the stroke—were all working in his favor. Dave had been very high-functioning in his former life, and so his brain had had an above-average number of neurons firing to do his work as an orthopedic surgeon. He had been fit and strong and highly engaged in a rich and complex life, full of family and friends and activity. These facts, coupled with his young age and his young brain's ability to regenerate itself, would be Dave's greatest assets. If he wanted to, they suspected, Dave would even be able to return to his residency as an orthopedic surgeon. They gave the target date of July 2016, one year in the future.

The room fell silent for a moment as we Levys looked at one another, a few of us with our mouths hanging open. We were elated, of course, but also slightly incredulous. The man I had just left in his room had to be told to drink the water that was in his glass. He could barely hold a pen steady enough to sign his name.

I believed in neuronal plasticity and I believed in Dave, but I also had the image freshly seared into my mind of Dave nearly dying. And then the reality that we had expected him to be in a vegetative state. Returning to orthopedic surgery? That was a line of work that I myself could never manage, and I've never had a stroke! And yet Dave would get back to that place?

This is what I wrote in my letter that night:

Dear Dave,

The family conference to get your prognosis was today.
They anticipate you making a full recovery.

Yay.

Wait, really?!?!?!?

YAY!!!!!!!!!!!

Yay, but how? You don't even know where you are. A full recovery? No really, how?

Chapter 26

THE TRANSITION FROM RIC TO HOME REALLY FRIGHTENED ME. RIC was a safe and contained cocoon, a controlled environment, while the real world was far from it. At RIC, I could be the supportive spouse and cheerleader, but the pressure of Dave's daily medical well-being did not rest squarely on my shoulders. Nurses monitored his vitals and made sure he took his pills and did not fall in the shower. His handful of attempts to shave himself had left him looking like an extra in the *Twilight* movies, but at least a legion of fantastic (and medically trained!) caregivers had been nearby to make sure he was not doing serious damage. Going home would be full of unknowns—suddenly everywhere I looked, I saw causes for alarm: staircases, front doors, car doors, a bathtub.

In some ways, our situation was more precarious than if Dave had been physically weaker. Because he was strong physically but not mentally, he was much more of a risk to himself. It was not unlike taking care of a toddler in the sense that we needed to do much of the thinking for him and keep him contained and safe— but our toddler weighed two hundred pounds. What if he decided to take a walk and ended up at the highway? Who would help him shower? Remind him to take his pills?

I was now in the third trimester of my pregnancy and on a tight deadline for my final book edits before the upcoming maternity leave. My agent had been a stalwart support and a faithful friend; my editor had been kind and understanding, as had everyone at my publishing house. I could have asked for an extension on the project and they would have supported me, but I needed to do this. For one, I had never in my life missed a deadline, and I'll be damned, I did not want to miss that one—the book was important to me, and I had worked really hard to get it ready for publication. And what's more, I wanted to get this book turned in before the baby arrived. As crazy as things already were, I knew they were only going to get crazier when a new little life joined our family. Currently, it felt like every moment of my day was devoted to taking care of Dave, but soon enough it would be devoted to taking care of Dave *and* a newborn. I needed to finish this book; I needed to do this for myself.

After several family powwows, we decided that Dave would transition to daily outpatient rehabilitation at the RIC branch in Northbrook, about thirty minutes north of Chicago. He would go through as intensive a program as was available—full days, five days a week. While he was there, we would live with Dave's parents.

I resisted this at first. I was about to bring a baby into the world and I wanted to be in my own home, not sleeping in Dave's high school bedroom. After the chaos of Fargo and the ICU and the inpatient stay at RIC, I was craving some return to normalcy. I was feeling the very real, biologically induced urge to set up my nest and prepare for the baby's arrival in my own space. And yet, Dave's parents made the very compelling case—and I came to agree—that I needed the support that would come from being surrounded by family.

Adjusting to our new normal in the northern suburbs, we settled into Dave's bedroom, surrounded by childhood sports trophies and high school photos. As truly lovely as my in-laws are, I was cognizant of the fact that I was in someone else's home. I was using someone else's kitchen and laundry room and bathroom. I was in someone else's space. And yet, if I had to be in someone else's home, I could not have asked for a better situation. My in-laws have always said: "The term 'in-law' is just a technicality; we love you like a daughter." They are family in all the best ways of the word, and they allowed us to feel completely at home.

There, in Dave's hometown an hour outside Chicago, we spent the last days of the worst summer of our lives. On the back porch, I edited my book to the sound of my father-in-law clipping the flowers. In the afternoons while Dave was at rehab, once I had finished working for the day, I would take the dog for a long walk or swim laps in a nearby friend's pool. My mother-in-law and I split cooking duties while Dave and his father split cleaning the dishes. At night, we would watch the birds at the bird feeder during dinner and then play a board game or cozy up on the couch and watch a television program before Dave's very early bedtime.

We took one very precious piece of cargo with us when we moved into the Levy family home. As we were preparing to leave RIC, I'd collected piles of letters and emails. So many of the people in Dave's life had been in touch regularly since the stroke, writing moving and heartfelt notes that Dave could not even begin to appreciate—at least not yet. I gathered up all of these notes that had come into our home and to his brother and to his parents. Letters from former teammates and college friends, people who came out of Dave's past to share stories of how he had inspired them or made an impact on their lives. My sister-in-law Erin bought a giant leather-bound book, and we put all of these letters into it, calling it "Dave's Book of Fan Mail."

Dave sat down on the couch and read this book on one of the first days we were back home. It took him several hours.

"What do you think?" I asked, watching as he leafed through the pages.

"I'm tired," Dave answered.

"Is it hard to read it?"

"Yes," he admitted, his voice faint. His body looked deflated. He was moved by these letters, but reading them took a lot out of him. He did not feel like the man these people had known, the man these letters described.

I felt similarly conflicted. It was inspiring and touching to read these words, yes. And yet I had to admit that there was a part of me that grew sad as well; all of these letters painted a picture of the man I had known and loved, a man who was no longer with us. I did not know if that man would ever come back.

Other things scared me, too. In fact, if I let it, worry could have wrapped its suffocating cord around me at all times. There was the time when Dave slipped going down the stairs and just barely grabbed the banister in time. The times when I would look over in the car and notice that he had not buckled himself in. There was the time when I did not like the look of a particular freckle and made him an immediate dermatologist appointment. I was petrified of losing Dave; I saw threats everywhere.

One day Dave and I took a walk in the evening when he got home from rehab. Before we had even taken a hundred steps from the driveway, Dave turned to me and told me he was dizzy; he felt that he was going to faint. We turned around and headed back inside and got him onto the couch before I went screaming through the house calling out for Dave's mother and father. "He's not having another stroke," Nelson told me, accurately perceiving the terror I was feeling. Dave was just dizzy from the bright sunlight and the heat and his eyes still being sensitive to so much stimulation.

I realized that this fear might be something I would carry around with me for the rest of my life, a vestigial scar from an injury that bore no outward marks. I decided then that I would never again wear the same flowy top and yoga pants combo I had been wearing on that fateful flight on June 9; I felt too strongly that to step back into those clothes would be to step back into those moments, first on the plane and then overnight in the Fargo ICU, and those were moments to which I wished never to return.

I knew that, going forward, my internal alarms would always be easily tripped, like when I made Dave uncomfortable by look-ing too closely into his eyes. "What are you doing?" he would ask, shifting under the intensity of my gaze. I was checking to make sure his pupils were not asymmetrically dilated.

While initially we had feared that they would require surgery, Dave's eyes gradually recovered on their own, with daily eye exer-cises that the neuro-optometrist assigned (we called them Dave's "eye push-ups"). One day at the neuro-optometrist's office, Dave had to put on a specific pair of glasses for one of his eye exams. They were funny-looking, with one lens colored red and the other lens colored blue. When Dave put them on he looked like a blend between Mike Ditka in his aviators and Elton John in his colored shades. I could not help but laugh, and Dave stole a glance at him-self in the mirror. "Oh, good lord!" Dave gasped, laughing at his own reflection. The reaction was so quick, so natural, so funny, so very *Dave*, I could not help but rejoice. He had seen himself and had noticed how ridiculous he looked, and had shown a self-awareness that I had not yet seen. I laughed, not only because my husband looked absurd, but also because he was aware of how absurd he looked and could laugh about it with me.

Slowly and with the daily exercises, Dave's cranial nerve recov-ered its functionality and his eyes began to self-correct. His up-and-down and side-to-side gazes returned, and his double vision decreased. Before long, double vision was a problem only first thing in the morning and in moments when he felt fatigued. And his eyesight bounced back, nearly to the 20/20 vision he'd had since his laser eye surgery. We were thrilled that Dave would not need to undergo corrective eye surgery.

One day something happened that caused even Dave to get a bit rattled. It was late September. He came downstairs from having done some brain exercises on a computer program called Lumosity. He sat down on the couch to read a newspaper. He noticed, as he was reading, that the words became jumbled. "I couldn't make sense of what I was reading," he would say later. "It was as if I could understand each individual word, one at a time, but I couldn't understand them all together in a sentence. I knew that something strange was going on; my brain felt weird."

After that, Dave felt drained and disoriented. He did then what he did so often when things were scary and overwhelming: he took a nap.

We call that "the event" because, aside from the stroke, it was the most significant moment for Dave. He felt like parts of his brain were literally firing up after being dormant. Like his brain was going through growing pains as it came grumbling back to life. "For me, it was confusing, but I knew it was a good thing because it meant that I still had neuroplasticity happening."

There were a few other moments like that when his brain "felt weird." He would complain of déjà vu or feeling disoriented. He felt, at times, like he knew what was going to happen before it did or that he knew what someone was going to say before he or she said it. These were all parts of his recovery and of the process by which his brain came back online.

So much of the brain and its functionality remains a mystery, a nebulous unknown, even to the experts, and the same applies to the recovery from a traumatic brain injury. It is not like rehabbing a broken bone or a replaced hip; recovery from a traumatic brain injury is not linear, and it is not an exact science. Sometimes things got a bit "weird"; sometimes things even felt like they got a bit worse before we could see a marked improvement. It was all part of the experience of a brain healing itself, and it was all a bit scary and at times distressing and at times encouraging. We had to cling to the hope that, even in the moments of chaos and confusion—perhaps *especially* in the moments of chaos and confusion—the healing was happening.

Chapter 27

Chicago, Illinois
June 2012

WHEN WE MOVED TO CHICAGO, I DECIDED IT WAS TIME TO SEE if I could seriously make a career of writing. I was so fortunate to be doing some part-time consulting work for the clean-energy company my father and some of his partners had started, and that work combined with Dave's modest salary as a resident was enough for us to live on. But flying back and forth between Chicago and New York was not sustainable for us, not if I wanted to really be a writer.

After years of flirting with the idea, after years of pursuing fiction in my off hours, I told myself I had six months to get a manuscript finished and into pitchable shape. I loved writing. It was all I wanted to do. But could I find a way to make it a career? Could I be a writer and actually have that support our life? I did not know.

I had spent the past four years sending my work to a literary agent, the fabulous Lacy Lynch at Dupree Miller & Associates, who had always been receptive and encouraging and supportive, but, just the month prior, her response to my entreaties had gone from "You're not ready for me yet, show me your next draft," to something to the effect of "All right, you are almost ready, let's do this."

We made our working relationship official in May 2012. We went from "dating to engaged," we joked, the month before Dave and I moved. I knew that Lacy could get my work onto the desks of interested editors—once my work was ready for that. I gave myself half a year to focus primarily on writing and pitching. If nothing came of it in that time, I would get a job selling yoga clothes or serving coffee and continue to pursue fiction on the side.

That summer I raced to finish up my manuscript of *The Traitor's Wife,* the historical novel I was working on about Peggy Shippen Arnold, the wife of Benedict Arnold and a significant character in his notorious treason during the American Revolution.

Dave was going through a rough adjustment to residency. He was feeling unsure of his skills as a surgeon and having a hard time getting comfortable in the hospital environment after so many years as a student. Plus, we were all on edge about Louisa, who was going through intense treatment for her multiple myeloma. That summer my mother-in-law underwent a stem cell transplant that took her to death's door. The procedure was horrific and the recovery was long and excruciating. There was a period of forced isolation when Louisa's body was too weak to be exposed to the germs of others.

After that treatment, slowly and steadily, under the loving and diligent care of her husband and loved ones and her outstanding medical team at the University of Chicago, Louisa grew stronger and began to feel better. Her hair began to grow back. She could eat and began to rebuild her muscles. A former triathlete, Louisa was not quite fully back to herself, but she was once again able to take long walks, so we enjoyed walking Penny together, talking about books and life and her excitement that she was going to become a grandmother for the first time as the air turned crisp and the colors of autumn began to touch the leaves.

By the fall, Dave and I were settling into some sort of rhythm in Chicago, but I was getting close to my self-imposed deadline to either jump into this writer thing full-time or make a responsible back-up plan to ensure that Dave and I would be financially stable during the years of his medical training.

I'll always remember the date: November 17, 2012. It was my mother's birthday, and I was flying out east for the Yale–Harvard football game, to be played that year at Harvard. Dave could not get off of work, so I was going to meet Marya and go with friends. When I landed in Boston, I turned my cellphone on. Immediately, it began to chirp at me.

I had a text message from Lacy, my literary agent: "**Can you talk?**"

A subsequent message repeated the same question, but with additional question marks. "**Can you talk???**" I also had a voicemail from Lacy. I listened to it.

Marya stood by the curb, waiting for me outside the airport. When I saw her, I was still listening to Lacy's voicemail, so I smiled at her, gestured that it would only be a minute more. I listened to the end of the message and hung up the phone.

I turned to Marya with a smile. How perfect that it was Marya—my former roommate and the first friend who had ever read my fiction, the first person to tell me that I could do it. "Mar, I sold my book," I said, incredulous. "Simon & Schuster is going to publish *The Traitor's Wife*."

Chapter 28

AS DAVE CONTINUED TO EXCEL IN PT, HIS INCREDIBLE RIC therapy team decided that we needed to come up with something to challenge and motivate him, something ambitious toward which he could work during sessions that might otherwise get boring. Exercise is beneficial for everyone, but for Dave, it was crucial for neuronal plasticity. All of the blood flow of the movement and exercise was good for Dave's brain as it worked to rebuild neurons. Plus, it was good for him to work on balance, and exercise is always a mood lifter. So his physical therapists did exercises with him that targeted both his body and his mind; he would balance on a plank while also answering trivia questions about orthopedic surgery, for instance.

It became clear that the treadmill and ordinary PT exercises were getting old for Dave, so his lead physical therapist, Liza, proposed that he train for a race in downtown Chicago called the Ditka Dash, named after the colorful Chicago Bears football coach Mike Ditka.

When Liza called me to suggest that Dave sign up for the race, I looked at the calendar with some concern. First, the race was less than a week before my due date. If I went into labor early—a distinct likelihood given how big I was measuring—then Dave would have to forgo the race. That was a small matter compared to my second concern: Was Dave ready for this? October would be just four months out from a stroke that had nearly killed him. He was weakened by the stroke and by his extended stays in several hospitals. In September, we had gone back into the hospital for a procedure on Dave's heart, during which they had closed his PFO, the hole that had likely contributed to the stroke. Long periods of bed rest and inactivity had sapped his strength.

Plus, Dave still fatigued so easily. A 5K would have been nothing for him before the stroke—he could have hopped it on one foot—but if he wasn't able to do it now, would he be disappointed in himself? Were we setting him up for defeat?

Dave agreed to do the race and began to train. He worked his way up from fatiguing after just a short walk to taking brisk walks on an incline to eventually jogging for a few minutes at a time on the treadmill. September turned to October. My belly grew bigger as Dave continued to train.

The day of the race was gray and chilly. Dave and I had stayed in our apartment downtown the night before—Dave's first time sleeping there. We drove over to Soldier Field, home of the Chicago Bears, early that morning for the race.

Everyone running in the race was invited to show up in his or her finest Mike Ditka attire, so, naturally, we were equipped. Dave wore a vintage Bears sweater that I had found for him on eBay one year as a Christmas gift. He had planned ahead (evidence of some executive functionality!) and had grown enough facial hair to give himself a cheesy Mike Ditka mustache. He paired those lovely details with aviator sunglasses and a sweatband around his forehead, and it was actually quite disturbing how much he resembled Ditka.

Dave's entire team of therapists showed up to run with him.

That they were all there so early on a cold, rainy Saturday morning shows just how dedicated they were to Dave, not only as a patient but as a person.

Dave's brother Mike had also signed up to run the race with him. Mike had not run much since a knee injury had required multiple surgeries years earlier, but he wanted to do this with his younger brother. We joked about who was worse off: the stroke patient or the guy with the bum knee.

Dave's parents were there for the race, as was Mike's wife, Marie, who was herself seven months pregnant and also toting around their fourteen-month-old. Marie and I waddled along, watching the runners go by. We made our way to the finish line and awaited Dave and Mike. We spotted them about twenty-four minutes later at the finish line. They ran by, big smiles under gross Ditka mustaches. Dave looked absolutely ridiculous, but he looked happy. His cheeks were flushed, and a sheen of sweat and October drizzle slicked his rosy skin. He had run the whole way.

I think I was happier than Dave was that he completed that race. I had wanted him to cross that finish line. *Now,* I thought, *we are ready to have this baby.*

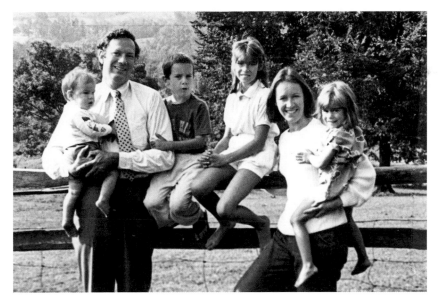

Alli is the third of the four Pataki siblings. From left: brother Owen; father, George; brother Teddy; sister, Emily; mom, Libby; and Alli in upstate New York. The family often spent portions of August in the area while George, then a New York state assemblyman, was in session in nearby Albany.

Dave is the youngest of the six Levy brothers.
Clockwise from left: brothers Jonathan, Erik, Scott; father, Nelson; mother, Louisa; brothers Mike, Dave, and Andy.
(Dave is the little boy in front in the denim jumpsuit.)

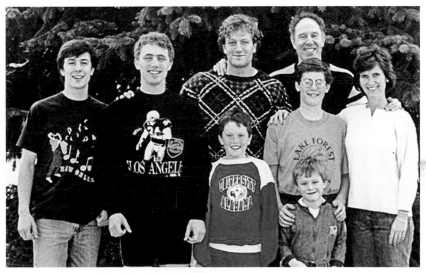

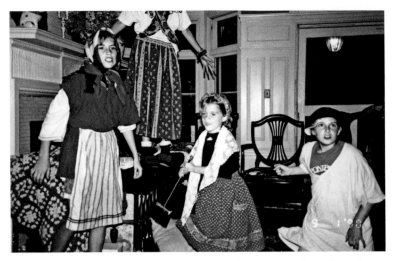

An early love of history and drama: Alli (center) plays the role of Cosette alongside her big sister, Emily, and friends in a living room production of *Les Misérables* at the Pataki home.

Dave lost his hearing as a baby due to a series of ear infections. He eventually regained it following surgery, but had missed eighteen critical months of cognitive development, necessitating hard work and intense corrective rehabilitation as a child.

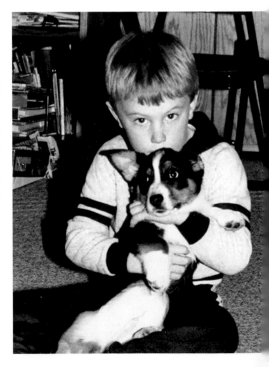

Salad days. Dave and Alli began dating in the fall of their sophomore year of college, though they had met in their first days as freshmen.

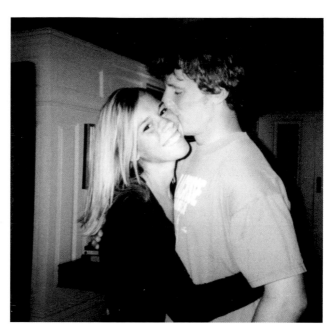

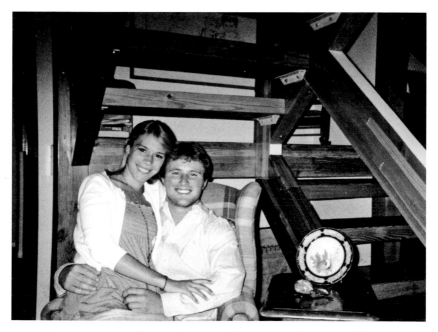

Summer 2005: Alli goes home with Dave to Lake Forest, Illinois, to see his hometown and visit his family and friends. Here they are sitting in the "chaperone chair" that Nelson and Louisa put outside Alli's bedroom.

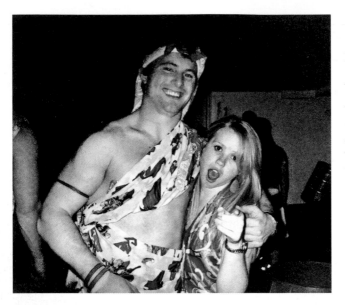

Dave and Marya (called "Mar Mar" by Dave) at a college toga party. Marya introduced Alli to Dave and was ever-present throughout much of their courtship.

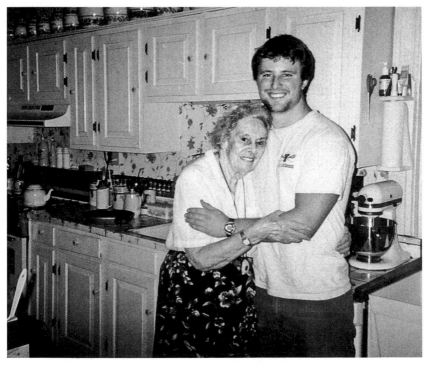

"Take a picture of us," Grandma Peg said as she took a break from frying eggs to hug Dave. She was the "first Pataki to make me feel like a member of the family," Dave says of Alli's grandmother.

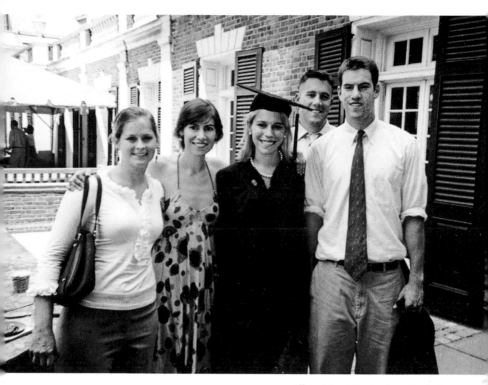

Alli with sister-in-law Emled;
sister, Emily; and brothers,
Teddy and Owen, on her college
graduation day, May 2007.

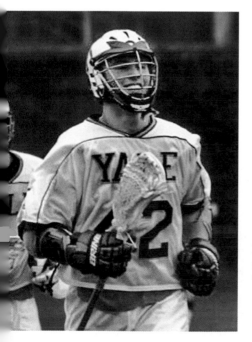

Dave as a starting
defensive midfielder for the
Yale Bulldogs lacrosse team.

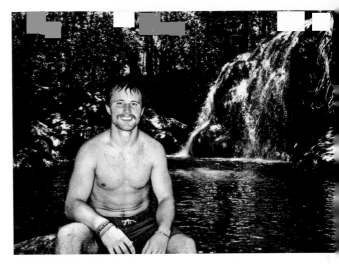

Dave traveled to Central America the summer between his first and second years of medical school to work in a clinic in Guatemala and study Spanish. Here, on a day off, he enjoys a hike and a swim.

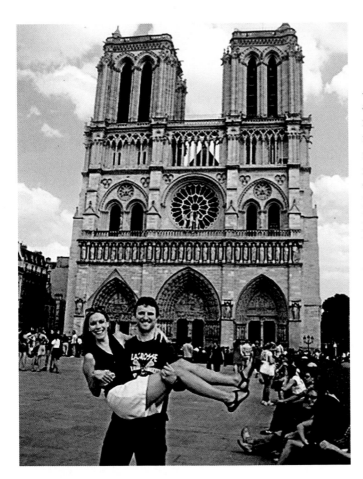

Alli quit her job as a news writer and moved to Paris for a few months, before returning to try to make a career of writing fiction. Dave visited in late June 2010; here they visit Notre Dame cathedral.

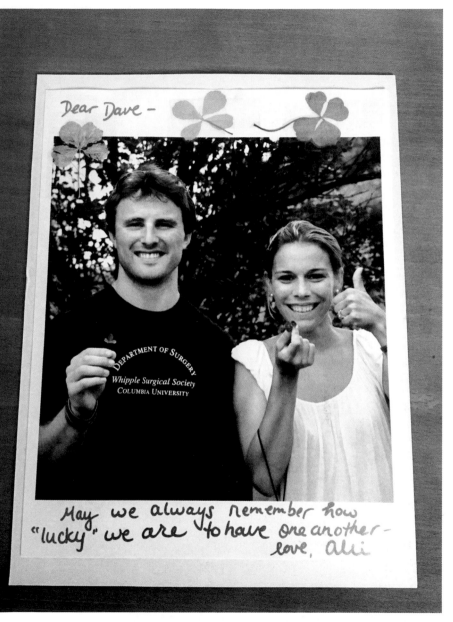

Dave and Alli got engaged in August 2010 at the Pataki family farm in
upstate New York. The next day, they found three four-leaf clovers;
Alli pressed them to give to Dave on their wedding day
with this note and picture.

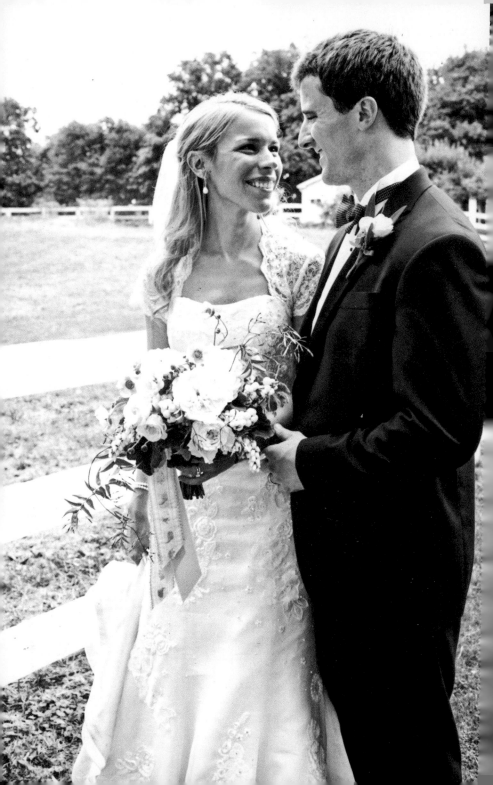

Dave and Alli were married in late September 2011, seven years to the day after their first kiss.

←

Dave graduated from Columbia Medical School in 2012, a day of mixed emotions: Dr. Nelson Levy flew out to New York City to watch his youngest son realize his dream of becoming a doctor, while Louisa, recently diagnosed with multiple myeloma cancer, could not travel from Chicago.

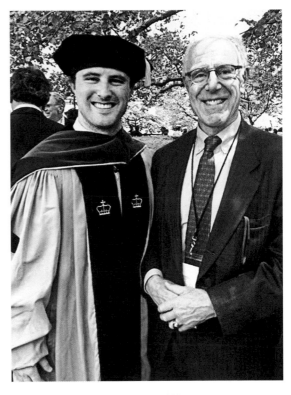

Members of the Levy and Pataki families gather at the Levy home outside Chicago for Thanksgiving 2012.

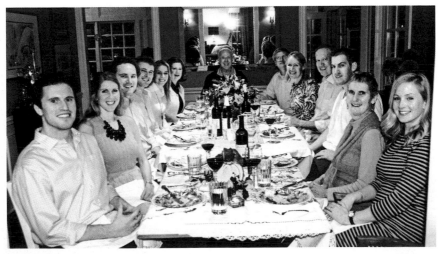

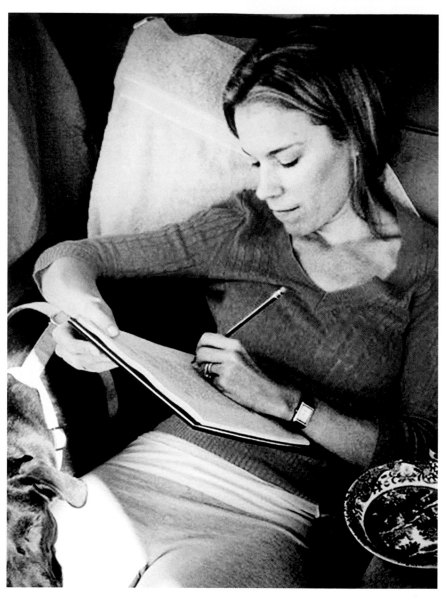

Alli works on the final edits of her first novel, *The Traitor's Wife,*
on the porch of their first apartment in Chicago.

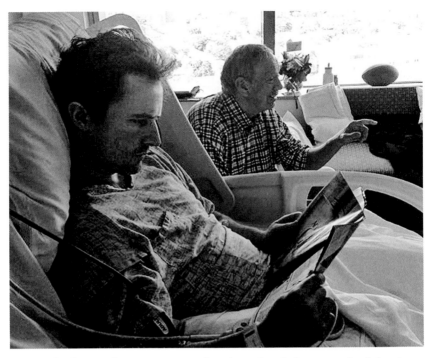

The early days in the ICU. Dave is disoriented and sleeps much of the time, surrounded by family and doctors. Here, he tries to read.

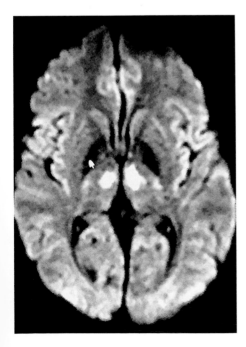

Magnetic resonance image (MRI) of Dave's brain on June 10, 2015. The clear white areas near the middle of the brain are infarcts (dead tissue) in both the right and left sides of the medial thalamus. The thalamus is the brain's major relay center, through which run vital connections between many different parts of the brain. Dave's brain had, in effect, two big holes of dead neurons at its center.

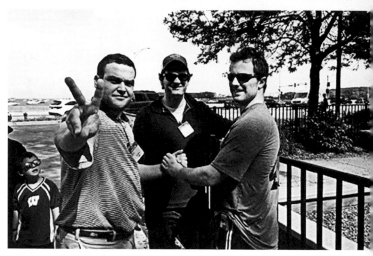

Dave's first memory after emerging from a state of amnesia
is this day with his best college friends Peter and Russell,
walking along Lake Michigan.

Friends Margaret and Charlotte made so many trips to
Target to stock Alli and Dave's new apartment that
the staff let them take a shopping cart home.

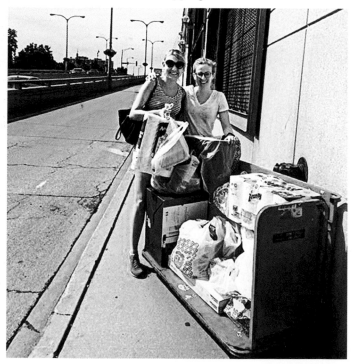

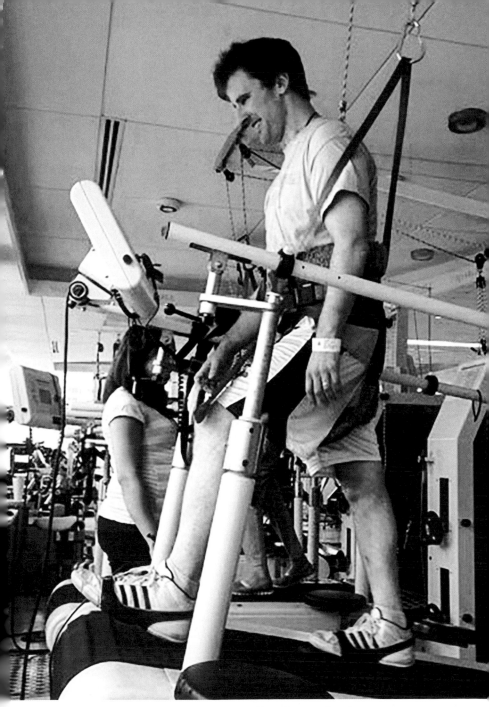

Dave could not walk on the treadmill without safety harnesses,
due to a lack of balance. He fatigued easily and was not at the level of
his former athletic self, but he enjoyed physical therapy.

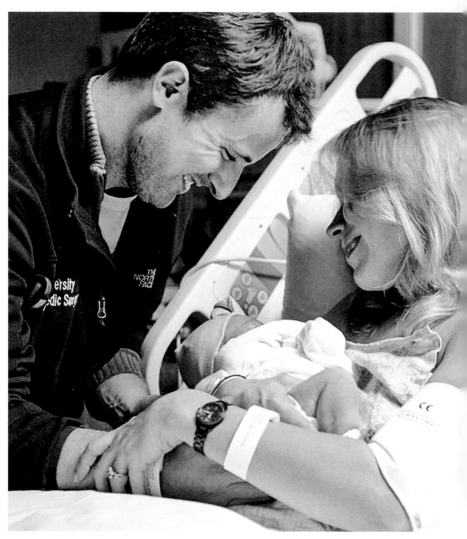

"I suspect that Dave will be able to participate in the birth of your daughter." That was what Dr. Richard Harvey told Alli, and she didn't believe it—but it turned out to be true when Lilly arrived in October 2015.

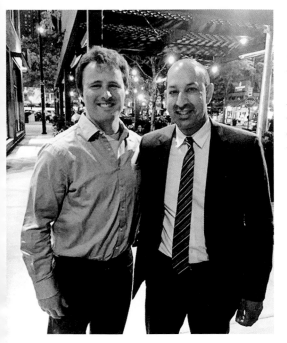

Dave with Dr. Omar Lateef, advocate, friend, and surrogate family member. Alli and Dave owed Omar cheeseburgers, as they'd originally agreed, but they went out for steaks instead.

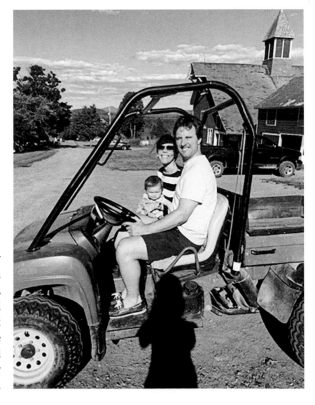

Just over a year after the stroke, on Father's Day 2016, Dave and Alli traveled with Lilly back to the spot where they became engaged. They found another four-leaf clover on that visit.

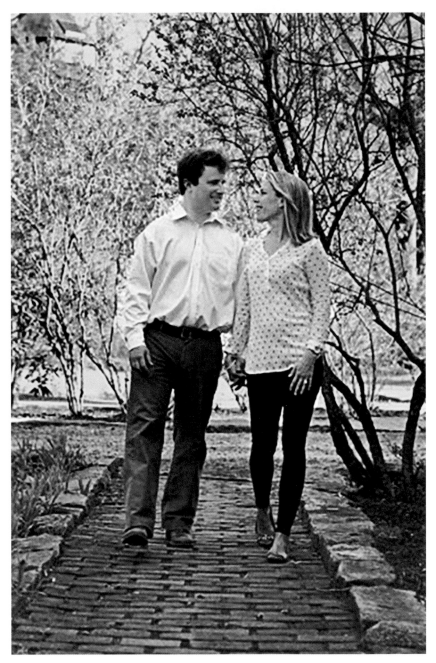

Dave and Alli, still holding hands,
still walking forward on the path together.

Chapter 29

Our due date, a Monday, came and went—so much for going into labor early. Five days later, on a Saturday, I awoke in the middle of the night with back pain. I had heard from everyone that early contractions felt like intense lower abdominal cramps, so it did not occur to me until about six A.M. that this back pain was coming and going in regular intervals and that I might in fact be having back labor.

We hung out that morning at home, waiting to see if this was the real thing or not. When I had to stop our pancake breakfast every few minutes to contort and writhe, hands pressing to my lower back, we decided that it was in fact real. Since Dave was not able to drive, my mother-in-law drove us down to Northwestern Prentice Women's Hospital, and we were admitted to the labor and delivery floor by midday.

Our baby girl was in no rush. The epidural worked its magic as I had contractions all day, FaceTiming with relatives and trying to wrap my head around the fact that we were about to become parents.

The Chicago Cubs were playing that evening for a chance to go to the World Series. It would be their first time playing in the World Series since World War II. They had not won a World Series in *over a century*. That they might now be on the verge of going to the World Series was a big deal; I cannot overstate how momentous this was for Dave and indeed for all long-suffering Cubs fans. The entire city of Chicago was in a postseason tizzy of red and blue. Our labor and delivery nurse told us: "I just moved to Chicago and I wasn't a Cubs fan, but now I am!" We put the game on in the background in our hospital room, Dave turning his attention toward the TV in between contractions.

The sun set on a beautiful fall day. Night fell over an entire city watching a baseball game. My baby was still taking her time, but finally, by nine, it was time to start pushing.

Our incredible rehab doctor at RIC, Dr. Harvey, had told us on Dave's first day there: "I suspect that Dave will be able to participate in the birth of your daughter." I had not really believed him at the time. Sure, I had wanted to believe, I had *hoped* that he was correct, but at the time I had doubts; I just could not see how Dave would be in any shape to participate in the birth, much less the tasks of caring for a newborn.

But he did, he was. Dr. Harvey had been correct. Dave sat by my side the entire time. He monitored my contractions, he cheered me on, and he brought me damp washcloths to swab the sweat from my face.

At one point, the nurse's attention was pulled to something across the hospital room and Dave jumped right in, counting down for me as I pushed through a contraction. The Cubs lost. It was an ugly defeat that, on any other night, would have crushed Dave, but on this night it was an afterthought.

After two hours of pushing, Lilly emerged and was there in the room with us; a part of this world, a part of our family.

It was not until a few weeks after the birth that my father-in-law admitted to me how nervous he and Louisa had been through the late months of my pregnancy and indeed throughout my labor (they sat in the waiting room for the entire day and night). They had been deeply concerned that the stress of the stroke and recovery might have had some adverse consequences on Lilly's health in the womb.

But when Lilly came out, she was perfect. I remember those first few moments so well: Lilly's first cry, the medical team clamping the cord and allowing Dave to cut it, the doctor and nurses whisking her across the room to the scale. Lying in the hospital bed, I watched, unable to rise and participate in the huddle around the baby, but I remember seeing Dave as part of it all, leaning over the scale, his eyes fixed on Lilly's soft, pink little body. I saw it in his face: he was completely smitten.

I thanked God for Lilly. And then I thanked God for the fact that Dave was there with us, that my daughter would know her father.

Chapter 30

Chicago

Winter 2013

Let's just say this: residency is a trying time for a marriage.

There were half a dozen other wives whose husbands were going through the orthopedic surgery residency with Dave. We called ourselves "the Rush Widows." These women understood how much it absolutely sucked, but no one else really could. I cannot tell you how often I heard some variation of the refrain from my friends and family whose husbands were not in medicine: "I could never do it!" or "I could never be married to a doctor!"

Well, I'd think, *I don't really have a choice, do I? The man I fell in love with happened to choose medicine—surgery—as his career, so I either leave him or go along for this difficult ride.* So there we were. And it was definitely a difficult ride.

I realize that there are many difficult and even dangerous jobs out there. I have two brothers who have deployed to combat zones with the military, so I realize that there are jobs in which men and women put their lives on the line every single day. I also realize that there are many, *many* people in this country who struggle to find work and to feed themselves and their families, and that a surgeon in a white coat is not a member of society likely to earn anyone's sympathy. I acknowledge and respect that, and I do recognize that once the training is done, orthopedic surgeons are more than generously compensated for their work.

But I do believe that medicine deserves its place in the pantheon of highly difficult jobs, particularly during the training years and particularly when you consider the strain it puts on the family balance. The length and rigors of training alone would send most sane people running for the hills: there are four years of premed courses, then the Medical College Admission Test (MCAT), then four years of medical school, then for most people a few years for research or private-sector work to round out their résumé at some point in there, then a five-year residency (give or take), and then a fellowship or two *after that*. While the rest of the people with whom you graduated from college are likely focusing on first jobs and then making their ways up in their careers and salaries, medical students remain in school and in training—very difficult school and training—for their entire twenties and then some. All the while they are getting paid an offensively low salary (if they're getting paid at all—for many of those years, they are *paying* exorbitant sums for training and schooling; many medical trainees begin their careers with hundreds of thousands of dollars of debt). The schedule and the lifestyle are punishing; Dave once computed what his residency pay came out to when his salary was distributed across the many hours he worked, and it was well below minimum wage.

Then there's the culture. The institutional ethos of so many senior doctors is, "Well, when *I* went through it, it was so much harder, so you should have to go through it, too." Doctors in training are junior members of the team, dues-paying underlings on the lowest rungs of the totem pole *well into their mid-thirties,* and that's if they take no time off between college and medical school.

Then there's the stress. I remember in the newsroom, the refrain we often used to calm ourselves when it got really hectic was: "We're reporting news here, not saving lives." But Dave could never fall back on that refrain because, well, he was tasked with saving lives. If I made a mistake at my stressful job in the newsroom, a typo slipped through onto live television. If Dave made a mistake at his job in the hospital, a life hung in the balance. That kind of pressure cannot help but weigh on you day in, day out.

Physically, Dave held up a lot better than I would have in his place. He would roll out of bed fifteen minutes before he had to leave for the hospital. He usually got no breakfast or lunch; dinner was often cold leftovers after I was fast asleep. He fueled his body with energy drinks and coffee. He was perennially dehydrated (which was sort of a good thing—he would not have had time to run to the bathroom on many days, anyway). Chronic sleep-deprivation was the norm. I remember one day when Dave woke up with the shakes and a fever of 103.9 and he still insisted on going into work. I remember thinking: *What about this situation is OK?* I often wondered why doctors are expected to take care of everyone else's well-being, yet they are not ever allowed to think of their own. It felt, at times, not only nonsensical but unconscionable.

A phrase that I once heard has stuck with me: *Medicine makes a most demanding mistress.* That is what it feels like so much of the time. When you are married to a doctor, you are sharing your spouse. Your time together is not your own. The pager goes off at all times—holidays, weekends, the middle of the night. You thought you could go home to see family for Christmas? Ha! You thought you could celebrate your anniversary? Rookie mistake!

Oh, and that wedding you wanted to go to—the one in which your *wife's sister* is getting married? Yeah, well, it depends on whether we have a case that day. There's a reason why the divorce rate among doctors is so high. It's so much more than a job. As the late Dr. Paul Kalanithi wrote, "You can't see [medicine] as a job, because if it's a job, it's one of the worst jobs there is."

It's got to be a vocation, a calling, the work for which you are willing to sacrifice so much else. Dave believed that if he could only make it to the other side of this grueling training, his work as a surgeon would always be something in which he could feel a deep sense of purpose and fulfillment—he was giving someone not just a new hip or a new shoulder, but a renewed ability to live life to the fullest.

But the years of training are trying.

All of those years, I could not help but look at my life and see the ways in which Dave and I were being, well, ripped off. How I was being short-changed as his wife. There were long hours logged at home alone. My friends could enjoy their weekends, could bring their spouses to weddings, could exchange Christmas presents on Christmas morning. Even on the few Christmases when Dave *was* home, he was not really able to enjoy it, being so tired or still fielding emails or pages or the threat of being called in at a second's notice. True, some of the other nonmedical professionals I knew worked as hard when they were on a specific project or account or case, but eventually the case ended, and usually brought with it sizable financial compensation. The stock market closes on holidays, legal cases eventually get resolved, schools close for the summer—but people never stop needing doctors.

I did not always excel in acknowledging how difficult it was for Dave. I am human and I wanted my husband around. I thought that having moved to his hometown for him awarded me some appreciation. He told me over and over again that I was his priority, but it often did not feel that way. And I often reminded him that that was the case.

And the stress and the lack of sleep got to him. How could it not? Being that perennially tired and overworked will take a toll on any personality. One midwinter night in his second year, Dave's car died at the hospital, after many long hours of being parked in the well-below-freezing temperatures while he remained inside, working a never-ending series of cases. Dave called me, his voice tired and stressed, telling me I needed to drive my car over to the hospital so he could jump-start his car. I was in my pajamas ready to get in bed, so this was not a call I was thrilled to get. I pulled on my snow boots, threw my heaviest down coat on over my pajamas, and headed out. When I got to the hospital, we hooked up the jumper cables. Dave's car sputtered to life, and my car promptly died. Dave and I were cold and tired and frustrated, and neither one of us was in a good mood. I remember thinking just how un-fun it all was.

Dave and I have always written back and forth to each other—hard copies of letters, little notes on a big day, emails, texts, and so on. My favorite aspect of Dave's gift to me on holidays is usually the card, because he always takes the time to write a long and thoughtful note. I cannot tell you how often during those years of residency my notes from Dave had some variation of the following:

> *I am so sorry that this has been so hard for us . . .*
> *It is especially when things are so difficult . . .*
> *Thank you for staying . . .*
> *This is so hard . . .*
> *I am so sorry . . .*

Dave considered quitting, on several occasions. They all do—that's something I learned from every single other wife I spoke with. They all go through those valley moments when it just does not feel like it is worth it. But Dave stuck with it. Dave has never been a quitter.

But you know what else he's not? A good bluffer. And that was another challenge he faced. A senior surgeon once told Dave that he needed to "work on his poker face." Dave was far too earnest, far too quick to reveal when he did not understand or agree with something. Maybe it's the politician's blood in me, but I generally have an easier time navigating murky social situations. I can put on a good face and work within most interpersonal dynamics. Dave cannot. There is no guile in him. It's both his best quality and at times his most crippling handicap. It's a plus that he's so honest and pure and genuine—one never wonders where Dave stands—but it can be a major handicap in a work environment filled with big personalities, opinions, and egos.

I remember one time in medical school, a few of the savvier students had started a trend of baking cookies for senior attendings. Dave thought this was an egregious and transparent display of kissing up. Dave is not much of a baker, so I offered to bake cookies that he could take into the hospital, but he flatly refused. We went to his parents' home and told this story to his brother, Andy, who was also in medical school at the time. Andy smiled and shrugged. "I baked cupcakes and brought them in."

"You *did*?" The disbelief was evident in Dave's voice.

"Heck, yeah, I did!" Andy said proudly, no trace of regret in his tone. "You've got to play the game."

This was a game that Dave did not know how to play very well. Dave's just not an adept horn-tooter; he's not a savvy self-promoter.

Writing, in large part, got me through those tough early years of residency when my husband was often gone or else home but tired or stressed or agonizing over something—a deadline, an upcoming surgical case, an unhappy higher-up, a research paper. I do not know how I would have coped if I had not had something to do at home that I loved so much. When I slipped into my writing groove, the hours flew by. I was incredibly productive those first few years of Dave's residency. I finished *The Traitor's Wife* and wrote *The Accidental Empress* and *Sisi* and several other manuscripts, along with scores of articles and blogs and guest pieces. Left at home with my imaginary characters, I was free from distractions, free to play and create and research and pour myself into not only writing but launching my career as a writer. I felt guilty at times that I loved my job so much and was able to do it at home in yoga pants while Dave was so miserable at the hospital.

When I ran out of steam and needed a break from writing, I would explore Chicago or go to yoga or meet up with girlfriends or my sisters-in-law or walk my dog. Penny, my daily companion, was another invaluable source of comfort during those years.

When Dave had long shifts or rotations at a hospital out of town, I would decamp to my in-laws' place in the suburbs. I had gone from being surrounded by friends, near my parents, near my sister, near my family's home, near my hometown where it was not possible to drive to the market without seeing ten people who had known me since childhood, to being seven hundred miles away from all of that, and with a husband who was often depressed or completely unavailable. And I struggled with that. But the Levys were so welcoming and loving that their place became a second home for me.

At that point Andy was the equivalent year to Dave in his own residency, and he was weathering many of the same challenges and frustrations. Andy and Dave would commiserate, and so would Erin and I.

I remember hearing that Avicii song, the dance hit with the lyrics *"So wake me up when it's all over. / When I'm wiser and I'm older."* I pulled out my phone and sent a text message to Erin.

"I feel like this should be our theme song during residency. Just wake me up when it's all over."

If Dave was not going to quit—and believe me, I reminded him countless times that that was an option—then there was nothing we could do but keep moving forward. We just had to get through it, together, taking refuge in the belief that it would someday get better.

Chapter 31

EVERY OTHER YEAR, THE HARVARD–YALE GAME IS PLAYED AT Yale, and Dave and I meet friends and family on the East Coast, where we go to the game and then stay in New York for Thanksgiving with my family.

At five months out from the stroke, November marked our first time flying with Lilly, and Dave's first time flying since that horrible June night.

When I booked the flights in October I was deeply concerned—would it be too difficult, flying with both a five-week-old and Dave?

But, by November, Dave had improved enough that, rather than adding to my list of concerns, he could help me with the baby, getting her and all of the luggage and baby gear through security and onto the plane. Because his stroke had occurred on a plane, I was having some jitters, reliving the horrible memories. I checked the pupils of Dave's eyes several times in the air to make sure there was not any asymmetrical dilation going on. He wore Lilly in a baby carrier for much of the flight, and the ride was smooth in every sense of the word.

We drove to New Haven for the game and were surrounded by loved ones in what is one of our favorite places on earth. Many close friends had visited Chicago and had an idea of the progress Dave had made, but other friends were seeing us for the first time since the stroke, and they all gave Dave big hugs and expressed their relief at how well he was doing. Lilly napped for most of the afternoon as she was passed from arm to arm. Dave had a beer at the tailgate—his first beer since the stroke. It was a sunny, chilly New England fall day, like so many other football games that we had enjoyed together over our eleven years as a couple. I thought many times throughout the day how grateful I was that Dave was there to enjoy it with us.

That night we went to one of New Haven's iconic restaurants, Mory's. The college tradition is to order big "Mory's Cups," large silver chalices that you pass around a big table, each person making a toast before taking a sip of the punch. We all made toasts; Dave's was a bit shaky, a combination of goofiness and a genuine expression of his love for our new daughter. We laughed over past memories and shared our joy in the fact that Dave was there.

I knew how long a road we still had. I knew that, in so many ways, Dave still was not himself, certainly not the indomitable version of himself that had once thrived on this campus. A dear friend admitted as much to me, saying, "People keep commenting how great it is to see Dave doing so well, but I think people who don't really know him that well don't realize that he's still not the old Dave." She was correct.

That's the thing about brain injury—it's invisible. Dave looked like his old self, and so people who saw him would breathe a sigh of relief and say how great it was to see him, back to himself. Dave did not bear any scars, did not walk on crutches, showed no outward signs to testify to the wound from which he was very much still healing. It was like the time a work colleague of mine inquired after Dave on a phone call, asking: "Where is he right now?"

"At rehab," I answered.

"How does he get to rehab?" this colleague asked.

"A car," I said. "Someone has to drive him."

"But . . . how does he get into the car?"

"He walks," I said.

"Oh! He can walk! That's great, I had no idea he was doing so well."

Throughout Harvard–Yale weekend, that was the common refrain: an expression of relief and happiness to see Dave doing so well. Back to his old self.

We knew, however, how far he was from his old self. He could walk, yes. He looked like himself, yes. But that had never really been the issue—at least not since the earliest days in the ICU when he had recovered much of his motor ability. Others could not see Dave's brain, could not understand that Dave's injury was not physical so much as it was cognitive and behavioral. Others did not know, as I knew, how easily Dave still fatigued and how much sleep he still needed. How passive he was at times, unable to make a decision or initiate an action or remember a scheduled appointment. That he still struggled to remember formerly easy things, like the content of a recent conversation or a new acquaintance's name. That he still found it challenging to do something as simple and seemingly second nature as log in to his online bank account or respond to an email.

But that weekend *did* remind us that we had cause to celebrate. That weekend, being surrounded by those who loved and rooted for Dave gave us hope for his continued recovery. Even just having Dave there, in that place where our love story began, was a cause for celebration. Had Dave died, that campus, the place of so much joy, would have become a place mired with heartbreaking memories. *How bright will seem through memory's haze, those happy, golden, bygone days.* So goes the Yale alma mater. Literally every corner of that campus and its surrounding city is redolent with memories of us. I would never have been able to go back without seeing the locations of our courtship, reliving the beautiful beginning of our shared journey. *But time and change shall not avail, to break the friendships formed at Yale.* It was true; we had not been broken. At least, not yet.

Chapter 32

NEITHER DAVE NOR I WAS NOSTALGIC ABOUT WISHING 2015
farewell.

We spent Christmas with Dave's family in Chicago, and New
Year's out east with my parents and our friends Charlotte and
Steve, who had a baby girl just five weeks younger than Lilly. As
four new parents, we did not even attempt to stay out until midnight on New Year's Eve; we hugged Charlotte and Steve good
night by nine P.M. and went our separate ways to carry out our
respective newborn bedtime routines. Once the baby was down,
Dave and I watched a movie and got into bed a few minutes before midnight, with Lilly sleeping in the next room.

"I'm so happy that this year is over," I told him as I clicked off
the light. I was ready to bid 2015 adieu, for sure. I asked Dave
what the highlight of his year had been. "Not dying," he answered.

"Huh." I whistled, releasing a slow exhale. "Yeah, I guess that's
about right." There was no topping that. I shut my eyes and
wrapped my arms tighter around Dave, giving thanks that I had
my husband beside me at the end of that year filled with so much
pain and beauty.

❖ ❖ ❖

When we got back from that New Year's trip, we moved out of Dave's parents' home in Lake Forest and into our apartment in downtown Chicago. The place that had served as a crash pad for me during the weeks that Dave was an inpatient—a lonely place to which I returned to sleep each night before going back to the hospital and rehab—had never felt like our home, and Dave had never even lived there, but it was time to officially move in. Dave had completed his outpatient therapy at RIC in the northern suburbs; he'd graduated out of physical and occupational therapy, and would now just be continuing with cognitive therapy a few times a week at the RIC campus downtown. Dave's parents were heading to their home in Florida for the winter; after six months of devoting their time and care to us, it was time for them to move forward. And we, as our small little family of three, had to move forward, too. To settle into our new normal.

It hit me hard. That first week we were back in January, the sky was dark gray and full of snow, and temperatures did not climb above single digits. Chicago's legendary wind is worthy of its formidable reputation; the ice-chilled air can cause physical pain to any parts of the body that are exposed. As venturing outdoors was not an option with a newborn baby, the three of us were stranded inside a new apartment that still felt unfamiliar. Because we had had to wait for the New Year for Dave's health benefits to replenish, we had not been able to schedule any upcoming outpatient therapy, and RIC in Chicago was booked solid through January. Dave would have a few hours of therapy all month, but the rest of the time it was up to me to stimulate him and fill his days.

In the first few months after the stroke, it had been easy for me to summon optimism and hope and energy. Nobody understood everything about Dave's injury or, therefore, his recovery. We had so many factors working in our favor and Dave woke up strong, so we had every reason to hope for the best. Setbacks in the beginning did not rattle me all that much—the stroke was still so recent, so fresh. I had the cool calm that comes from being in the eye of the hurricane (and perhaps even from being in a state of semi-shock); I had the blinders on that do not allow you to focus on anything other than the immediate needs of the crisis. All of that "This is a marathon, not a sprint" and "It'll be a long road" felt vague and theoretical; I was fresh out of the gate, surrounded by a constant circle of loved ones, and I still had the energy of the sprinter.

Several months out, setbacks still were not *that* scary. They could be brushed off as the expected bumps in the road that constitute traumatic-brain-injury recovery. I filed it all under the "Two steps forward, one step backward" and "It'll be a roller coaster" talk. I was living with my in-laws, we still had a ton of support around us, and I still had some reserves of energy and optimism. And while my body was growing ever more unwieldy, there was not yet a newborn baby to sap my time or focus or strength.

But here, alone, in the deep freeze of dark January, adjusting to life with a new baby and facing a new year—the year in which Dave had set the goal of returning to his demanding work as an orthopedic surgeon—it was troubling to see that many of Dave's deficits persisted; it was hard not to worry that these lingering deficits might in fact be here to stay, that they were predictive of where things might settle out. Perhaps we had gotten all the recovery we could expect. Perhaps we had reached the dreaded plateau. No one could tell us, because no one knew.

I noticed the deficits most glaringly in Dave's lack of motivation and initiation. The old Dave had routinely worked for more than fifteen hours a day, entirely of his own volition. How many times had I begged him to stop working at night or over the weekend or on vacation? No one had needed to light a fire under Dave

Levy. Now, however, Dave was lethargic and laid-back and entirely unlike his formerly Type A, overachieving self.

This was like some new, morphed, entirely unrecognizable version of the man I had known and loved. When I asked Dave's therapists about this, I learned that this apathy had to do with Dave's still-inadequate executive functioning.

Executive functioning is the last thing to develop in a mature brain. Most of us do not develop executive functioning until our early twenties, which is why teenagers are so often thoughtless, messy, forgetful, and in need of so much sleep. When I examine my own past, I can notice that there was in fact a marked difference between myself as a senior in college and a senior in high school. I had pegged it as a function of maturity and time, but I could now concede that, yes, this "executive functioning" I was hearing about must also have been a significant factor.

Dave had lost the higher functions of his brain and, with that, his executive functioning—his ability to be the self-starting, responsible manager of his own life as an adult. In the earliest days of his injury, Dave had resembled a newborn baby: entirely helpless, sleepy, lacking in all language, unable to perform the most basic of daily tasks. Then he had grown into an oversized toddler: impulsive, unpredictable, still helpless, but sweet. Now, after seven months of recovery, Dave's brain had matured enough to put him at about a teenager—my husband was now like some petulant, sleepy high school boy.

This was a tough place for us to be. He was lucid enough to resent my urgings (nagging, as he called it), but not sharp enough to initiate and take over all of his self-care. I struggled to navigate the dual roles of both wife and caregiver. I did not want to have to nag him, and I certainly did not want to argue with him over whether he needed my help.

Previously I had been patient and positive. I had rolled with the setbacks and known that we were still very much in the midst

of recovery. But now my patience began to fray as I acknowl-
edged that I did not know where this recovery would take us. Was
this going to be my life forever? Was this going to be my marriage forever?

I had a newborn baby to take care of, and I was physically,
emotionally, and mentally exhausted after months of nursing
both my husband and our baby. On the one hand, Lilly was a
dream infant—she was sleeping through the night and she was
healthy and happy and had a very easygoing disposition. In many
ways, we joked, she was the best-behaved member of our household. But, still, I was taking care of a newborn. That's a full-time
job, and that alone can make the days feel long and tedious, no
matter how much you adore your little one.

Plus, with the move back downtown, I had gone from having
the support and company of my in-laws to running a household
entirely on my own. I had no loving family member around to
whom I might hand the baby over if I absolutely needed a nap
or a shower or a quick mental break. Nelson and Louisa were
planning their relocation to Florida; Andy and his family had by
this time moved to Colorado for Andy's fellowship. Mike and his
family lived in a suburb about forty minutes outside of Chicago,
but they had two babies under one and a half and were understandably overwhelmed in their own busy lives.

With the end of the holiday season, I no longer had the company of my own family, either; I no longer had the frenzied distractions of reunions with friends and the frenetic busyness of
the happy holiday season. My parents and siblings and closest
friends were all at least seven hundred miles away. As we cleared
up the Christmas decorations and pulled out our heaviest winter
coats, I realized that I was suddenly very isolated and very much
alone with my baby and my teenager-like husband.

As we settled in for a long, cold, dark Chicago winter, I began
to see our new reality through a film of despair. I was lonely and

I was frustrated and I was pale and I was fed up and I was tired; "weary" is probably a better word.

And I was scared. Terrified. It was impossible to know which among these new characteristics of Dave's were here to stay, what was simply Dave's new permanent personality. *Our new normal.* If I'd had to put some number on it, I would say that Dave was 75 percent back to himself. And that was great—I knew we had so much to be grateful for. But that 25 percent was what had made Dave *Dave.* That was the part that had made him a unique man, *my* man, the man I loved. I didn't know if that 25 percent would ever return. I wept to Margaret over the phone: "I don't know if I'll ever get my husband back." Even though my husband was physically there, in the apartment, home every single day, I had never felt so alone.

Dave remained positive in his outlook—but even that, I worried, came from a lack of depth and understanding—a childlike and incomplete grasp of the grim realities surrounding him. He remained confident that he would meet the very high bar of resuming his work as a surgeon. Rush remained incredibly supportive of Dave and his goal to return to the residency. We met with Dave's residency program director, and she was adamant that Rush would make it work, that they would welcome him back into the program in the class one year behind his original class. Dave's mentor had issued an open invitation for Dave to shadow in his clinic as soon as he was ready to ease back into the hospital environment. They offered us support while also being respectful of the privacy and time that Dave needed to heal. They offered to let him attend conferences, participate in research, work in the scope labs, and do whatever else he needed to do to facilitate his transition and return.

And yet I worried that perhaps we were all deluding ourselves in thinking that Dave could return to such an arduous lifestyle. I wanted to be supportive and hopeful, to believe in my husband, but I also could not ignore the fact that he was sleeping fourteen hours a day. That he had to be reminded to take his keys with him when he left the apartment. How would he possibly get back to a place where he could operate on a living human?

Dave noted and received my frustrations with frustrations of his own. He countered that I had no idea how hard it was for him to simply get through the day. He reminded me that it was *he* who had suffered the stroke, not I, and so could I please stop acting like this was so hard for *me*? We had very difficult moments, and I was absolutely not surprised in the least when I heard that the divorce rate for couples going through traumatic brain injury was as much as three out of four. (Why do Dave and I always find ourselves in situations with such high divorce rates?) Dave was justified in feeling the way he felt, as I was justified in feeling the way I felt. There was no easy answer, no easy way to forge a path through the darkness.

Because the recovery from a traumatic brain injury is not linear, it will play awful games with your mind and your soul. One day Dave would be showing evidence of great progress; I would allow myself to feel tingles of hope, and to believe that perhaps we had turned a corner, and then the next day it would feel like Dave had taken huge strides backward. The best analogy I heard to make sense of the situation came from Lee Woodruff: "Traumatic-brain-injury recovery is like one of those freaky carnival fun-house mirrors, where the image shifts on you. One minute, things look almost normal, and then, all of a sudden, *boom!*, the image morphs on you, and everything is distorted and unrecognizable and downright frightening." Exactly.

There was something else that was weighing on me: I had a book launch coming up. After having two consecutive *New York Times* bestsellers, I had been so excited to launch *Sisi*. I loved this book, I felt a deep attachment to the characters in *Sisi* and the historical figure upon whom this novel was based, and I wanted to do her story justice. I had worked so hard to launch my career as an author. Would a flop at this crucial juncture send my entire career onto a downward trajectory? Would I be disappointing people—readers? my publisher? my agent? myself?—if I could not give this my all?

Book launch is a demanding and hectic time under the best of circumstances. My previous two launches had been chaotic whirlwinds, and I had had neither a newborn nor a husband recovering from a stroke with which to contend. Here, in my new reality—my Target pajamas stained with various bodily fluids from my newborn, struggling to make time for a cup of coffee or a shower while begging Dave to put a reminder in his iPhone to take his medications—I looked ahead with dread and panic.

"It will be good to have something else to focus on," a well-meaning friend said about the upcoming launch. "Something to look forward to. An opportunity to celebrate *you.*"

But I did not feel like being celebrated. I was just so tired. So very weary.

"My reality these days is wiping poopy diapers and attending rehab," I wept to Lacy one day over the phone. "How can I possibly pull it together for a book interview or a launch event?"

I was not certain that I could. I was not certain that I had it in me to get to the next day, the next diaper, the next rehab appointment, much less not break down in tears on national television. How could I sit there and smile and shake hands at some fancy book event when I had so many bigger things going on in my life that were draining my mental, physical, and emotional energy?

It was not about the glamorous book events or the chatty interviews, really. It was a reckoning on my part with my ability to keep moving forward in a life that now felt so scary and uncertain and entirely altered. It all felt so discordant, like a big fat lie—I did not want to make book-party small talk; I did not want to pretend in front of all of those people that I had it together and that things were good. *We're doing just great! I have it together! Want to read my book?* I was having a hard enough time just keeping myself together in front of my husband and my baby. There was no part of my show that I wanted to take on the road.

"You are in your ocean time," Lacy told me, switching gears from butt-kicking agent to compassionate confidante and loyal friend. When I asked her for clarification, she added, "You're out in the middle of the ocean. You're too far along on the journey to see the land behind you, the shore from which you left. But you're not close enough to see the land to which you will arrive. All you can see right now is the ocean, and all you have to go on at this point is faith. All you can do is keep swimming until you begin to see the outline of the next shore."

Could I keep swimming? Did I still believe that there *was* a shore in the far distance? Some place to which I could arrive and feel safe again? Perhaps even happy? I did not know.

Insomnia, my nemesis from past seasons of stress, returned. "Brain spin" is what my mom calls it; in spite of how exhausted I was, my mind would reel all night long with fear and anxiety. Lilly was sleeping like a dream—twelve hours a night—but I sure wasn't. Each morning, crawling out of bed and looking ahead to another long and excruciating day, I felt shakier than I had the day before.

I was suddenly rail-thin. People marveled, tossed out well-meaning compliments on how quickly and completely I had shed the baby weight. "What is your baby weight-loss secret?" they would ask. *Stress!* I would think. *It's remarkable, really, what stress will do for the waistline.*

I was so weary of hearing comments like "I could *never* do what you are doing" and "I don't know how you're doing it." Each comment like that, well-intentioned as it was, only seemed to shine a fresh spotlight on how undesirable my life and our circumstances were. It was like a compliment that highlighted the pain. I was also tired of hearing "We're worried about you" and "You can't do this alone."

If there had been a transcript for my thoughts when I heard remarks like that, it would have gone something like this: *First of all, I'm not "doing it," whatever you think "it" is that I'm doing. I'm barely coping. I'm getting through each day by fighting back tears and meltdowns, and then at night I thrash around in bed wrestling anxiety and fear and sadness and anger. But not sleep. Sleep is impossible, even though I need sleep. Even though I'm more exhausted than I could have ever imagined possible. So, please, don't commend me.*

Second, you could do it. Because it's not a choice. This stroke was foisted on my family. It's not like we chose it and then decided whether or not we could deal with it. We have to deal with it because it's our reality. And if it was your reality, you would have to deal with it, too. I don't ever wish this on you, but if you had to do it, you would have to do it, just like I have to do it. And OK, if you're worried about me, then pick up some groceries for me, or come over and hold my baby so I can take a shower or a nap. I'm not doing this alone by choice; I don't want to be alone. I'm asking for all the help I can. I need help. So any help you would like to offer would be appreciated. But don't tell me you're worried, because then, being the pleaser that I am, I will worry that you are worried. That shifts the burden onto me to now have to somehow reassure you that I'll be OK and that you can stop worrying. See how that happens? And I don't need that right now.

Fortunately, I never said any of that aloud, at least not in that raw of a delivery, but in some of my lower moments, that was how I felt.

Chapter 33

DAVE HAD ALWAYS BEEN THE ONE TO CHECK THE MAIL. IN OUR modern age of email and text messages and voicemail, I'd come to think of "snail mail" as largely irrelevant, a pile of twenty tedious pieces of paper—credit card solicitations, flyers announcing a new neighborhood pizza joint, bank statements that could just as easily live online—for every one piece of meaningful correspondence. And so, over the years, I'd willingly ceded that chore to him. It's not something we'd ever talked about or decided on, but as is so often the case in any relationship, we'd settled into our way of doing things, divvying up the minutia of our day-to-day life together. Dave didn't mind checking the mail, I did, so that was just something that fell in Dave's column—it was one of his things, the way taking out the garbage and washing the dishes were his things.

And so, that winter, as all of Dave's "things" shifted from his column into my already-packed column, checking the mail became yet another task to think about in order to keep our day-to-day life afloat. I resisted it at first. I dislike checking the mail on a good day, but in recent months—the stroke, emergency medical transports by land and by air, extended ICU and hospital stays at Fargo and Rush and RIC, dozens of doctor's appointments, therapy sessions, blood-clotting tests, scans of the heart and brain and pretty much everywhere else, medication lists, Dave's surgical heart procedure, a pregnancy, a delivery and subsequent hospital stay, a newborn baby with her own medical visits, and so much more—the act of sorting and responding to our family's mail had gone from inconvenient to outright harrowing.

It was piles and piles and piles of paperwork. Bills that felt like a fresh punch in the gut each time. Insurance fine print that was long and confounding, often filled with pushback that sent a new surge of fight-or-flight hormones churning through my already-hormone-addled body. Disability applications that required my time and attention. Doctor visit summaries and reminders for so many upcoming appointments. An application to get my breast pump reimbursed. Not to mention all of the paperwork that comes with getting a new life up and running: birth certificate application, Social Security registration, her own health insurance coverage, and neonatal appointments. As twisted as it sounds, even the well-wishes and baby gifts arriving in the mail from generous friends and family began to feel like a burden as I thought: *Unwrap another package, recycle the packaging, and then write another thank-you note.*

Each day it arrived, a never-ending barrage of crushing mail, more paper to add to the pile. I was so tired of it. I was tired of fielding these bills, figuring out which ones needed payment and which ones required me to call the insurance company and wait on some automated line until I finally got redirected to a person with whom I could argue (plead? cry? reason?) to get Dave the treatments he so desperately needed. My to-do list was already too long, but each piece of new mail inevitably meant some new chore, and it was I who would have to manage it.

My way of coping with this was, for a time, to simply stop

checking the mailbox altogether. Avoidance. Denial. Walk right past the building's mailroom and don't look in. If I didn't see the piles of paperwork, I didn't have to do the paperwork. Right?

So then one day, after about a week of not checking the mail, I skulked reluctantly into the mailroom, my tail between my legs, unhappily facing the reckoning. I slid the key in and opened our mail slot, bracing for the backlog. I looked in. Nothing. Empty. Not a single piece of paper. Not a single bill.

Hallelujah! I thought. *Halle-freaking-lujah! Maybe things are finally calming down? Maybe I'm finally getting a handle on things, maybe I've finally caught up on our piles of paperwork?* Not having mail was the single best thing that had happened to me all day.

"Oh, hi, miss?" Just then an attendant who worked the daytime shift of our building's lobby was peeking into the mailroom. "You're in apartment 201, right?"

"Yes," I answered.

"Your mailbox was overflowing. The postal carrier couldn't fit any more mail in, so he moved all of it."

"Moved it?" I asked, my giddy relief evaporating. "To where?"

"Here." The man handed me a sticky note. On it was an address. "This is the USPS processing facility for this part of Chicago. You'll have to go there and collect your mail."

I took the note, my stomach dropping. How fun it would be to take my infant out in the bitter cold to wait in line at a USPS processing facility in the hopes of finding piles of bills and other medical paperwork.

"You had a *lot* of mail," the man said after a moment, a friendly smile on his face.

"Yeah," I said. "We get a lot of mail."

"Probably best, then, to check it every day, so the mailbox doesn't overflow."

❖ ❖ ❖

Have you ever wanted to just trade lives? To say: *I can't do this anymore; can someone take over for me? Can someone else carry this for me, even just for a day?*

That was how I felt in some of the moments of the deepest dark. I was fried from tending to the baby while trying to stimulate Dave's brain and recovery while also keeping track of everything at home—keeping the fridge stocked and the prescriptions filled and the laundry clean and the car battery from freezing and the dog walked (even though it was single digits outside), all while trying to keep my own career afloat. And if Dave was not going to return to work, then hadn't I better begin seriously thinking about how I would become the primary breadwinner? It was not pretty.

What I needed was sleep, and support. I sent out an SOS message. My mother-in-law delayed her planned departure for Florida and stayed with us downtown for a week to help with the baby and Dave. She cooked us lasagna and rocked the baby to sleep and spent hours with Dave, diligently setting up his home office with him, approaching the tedious task with a patience and a calm that I simply no longer had in me. Louisa is like a talisman, one of those holy objects whose very presence in a room keeps the dark spirits at bay. With Louisa in our home, I felt a light and a love that I just did not have when we were home alone.

As Louisa left, my mom flew out to join us. She, too, is a bulwark, the rock-solid support I needed right then. She made me coffee in the mornings and held the baby so I could nap. She walked our dog and stocked our fridge. She brought a fresh energy and positive outlook into our small, struggling family circle. One of my favorite photos of Lilly is from that week my mom spent with us in Chicago in January: it's evening, and Dave is holding his daughter in his lap, smiling, while my mom looks on in the background, the loving grandmother holding her glass of red wine. The dark night outside the window does not appear as terrifying with my mom in the room, smiling, looking on.

After that, my aunt Christine came. She had not been to Chicago in years, and so she inspired us to get out and see the city. We went to museums and braved the cold to take walks. She cooked for us and opened up about the hard times in her own life, and we had a wonderful visit as she got to know Lilly. Marya came back, too. I just needed support and community and I needed my best friend, with whom I could be entirely raw. Every morning that Marya was there, I would stumble out into the living room, Lilly on my hip, and I would say: "I love waking up and knowing that you are here." I needed to feel like it was not all resting so squarely on my shoulders. I needed to feel like I could speak and have someone there to listen and to answer and to understand. One day, when our car was towed and then died at the tow lot and I had to trek out in the snow to go jump it and drive it back home, it came as no small relief that I could leave the baby at home, warm, with Marya.

There is one day that sticks in my memory. Dave and Lilly and I were driving to rehab in the morning. I had noticed that, since the stroke, Dave never answered his phone. And not just that—he never checked email, text messages, or voicemails. He just did not care. So, in the car that morning, I urged him to listen to his voicemails. "Oh," Dave said, listening to one of the recordings. "That was RIC. My rehab this morning is canceled."

I slammed on the brakes. "What? Why?"

"Not sure." Dave shrugged. "They didn't say."

"Play the message again," I insisted. "Put it on speaker."

Dave rolled his eyes but obliged. We listened to the message. They *did* say: the therapy was canceled because of some issue with insurance.

"When was that call?" I asked. "When is that voicemail from?"
Dave checked his phone. "A few days ago."

"Why don't you *ever* answer your phone?" I asked, my teeth
gritted. "Or listen to your voicemails?"

Dave shrugged again. "It's fine. No big deal. We'll just reschedule."

"No," I growled, "*I'll* reschedule. After *I* deal with whatever dispute this is with the insurance." I wanted to scream. Not only had
we gone to the trouble to load up the baby in frigid weather, arrange her nursing and naps around making this appointment,
and then driving through the snow to get Dave where he needed
to be. Not only had Dave's much-needed therapy been canceled
because of yet another frustrating insurance dispute. Now it
would fall on my shoulders to fix the issue and reschedule the
appointment. *But Dave had not even bothered to listen to the
voicemail.* Had he listened to the voicemail, perhaps we could
have resolved the insurance issue by now. Perhaps we could have
salvaged this appointment. At the very least, we would have been
spared the effort of loading us all and driving us all through the
snow to rehab.

And what was more, now that Dave had no therapy that day,
what were we going to do with him? Was it just another day of
arguing at home—Dave insisting he could nap and watch TV
while I nagged him to read or exercise or do *something* to stimulate his brain?

That night, Dave went out to dinner with his friend Brad. Evenings out like this with close guy friends were a welcome reprieve, both for Dave and for me. He could get out of the house
and away from me and my evident misery. And I could have a
few hours off, with only the baby, who was an easy keep compared to Dave.

That evening, as I was preparing Lilly for bed, changing her
diaper and getting her into her pajamas, I began to kiss her soft,

squishy skin. In that moment, I heard something I had never heard before: a beautiful, soul-lifting sound. My baby's first laugh. I froze. I realized that my kisses on her bare skin had tickled her and she had laughed. I looked at her, startled and delighted. It was the best sound I'd ever heard. I kissed her again, this time a bit more vigorously. She laughed again. I kissed her more, on her neck and her shoulders and her arms and her belly. Lilly erupted into peals of sweet, innocent, carefree laughter. I looked down at her with tears pooling in my eyes, crying and laughing over her at the same time. I took a video of these first laughs and sent it to both of the grandmas, my sister, and my sisters-in-law. Marie wrote back: **"Isn't it the best sound? An instant mood lifter."** It was true. As I watched Lilly there, laughing on her changing table, I thought: *How is it possible for my heart to hold such overwhelming feelings of joy and grief at the same time?*

After agonizing over it and doing a ton of research and speaking to a variety of well-informed sources in my life, I decided that I needed to try a low dose of antidepressant. "Body armor" was how one expert referred to it. My reserves were utterly depleted. My body and soul had been ravaged with the stress on me—the pregnancy, the delivery, taking care of a newborn, all while juggling Dave's stroke and recovery. I had days when I felt bereft of all hope, and I needed a safety net under me so that I could begin the hard work of pulling myself back up.

I leaned on my friends and my family; I made my need evident in a way that I had never done before. Never before had I been so tapped out, so painfully aware of my limitations. I had always been someone who had prided myself on having it more or less together. I had been the planner, the supporter, the self-sufficient one. I had been the one who listened quietly on the phone to a weeping friend or family member and offered advice or words of comfort. I had not been the one weeping into the phone. I could count on one hand the number of times, prior to those days, that I had wept to my parents. But this—this was beyond me.

I was crying a lot. Because my reserves were so utterly shot, I was quick to snap at Dave. He, understandably, was quick to snap back or, worse, retreat into defensive and silent seclusion. This, of course, only drove me to fresh bouts of fury.

One night in midwinter we had one such argument—I honestly cannot even remember what it was about. But I do remember that I got so mad and so upset about whatever it was he said to me that I picked up the phone and dialed Marya. I could not speak to Dave. I could not look at him. I wanted to ask him to leave the apartment, to kick him out, even though it was probably twelve degrees outside and he was a stroke patient and our infant daughter was sleeping in the next room.

I needed Marya to calm me down, talk me back from the precipice, and she was the right person to do so because she would not simply take my side, and I knew that. She loved me, but she also loved and understood Dave. I did not want to simply vent and rant to someone who would just agree with me, echoing my rage and indignation back to me. That would not be helpful. What I needed was to hear from someone who loved Dave, because I did not feel, in that moment, like I did.

As the phone rang I looked at the clock. Just past eleven in Chicago, after midnight in D.C. *Oh crap,* I thought. Her fiancé was going to think I was crazy, calling after midnight, crying into the phone.

Marya answered almost immediately. "Hello?"

"Mar. Hi. I'm so sorry—it's past midnight. Did I wake you?"

"No," she said. I'm not sure if she was lying. "What's up?"

"Marya, I don't want to be married to Dave anymore."

"OK." I heard her rearrange herself on the other end of the line, sitting up to attention as I bawled into the phone. "Want to tell me what's going on?"

I relayed to her the details of that night's fight. It was all more than I could bear. Not only did I resent that I had to nag Dave to do so many things, but I resented the fact that he resented my nagging. If he didn't want my help, then he could just get out and go figure this all out on his own, because God knows I did not want to be carrying his load anymore. "I just can't do this anymore," I moaned. "He says these things that are so offensive. After everything I'm doing for him! Or worse, he'll say these things that are just completely nonsensical and irrational. I can't even talk to him. I can't look at him."

"OK," Marya said, her voice calm. "Alli, you need to remember something: Dave had a massive stroke a few months ago. His brain is not entirely healed. He is not entirely himself. Do you *know* how fast you speak? Do you *know* how much you throw at him when you get fired up? His brain can't keep up. I'm sure when you get mad at him and start laying it all out before him, he gets confused and scared and of course he gets defensive. So then he just says something back so that he can defend himself, but it might not make sense, and it might not follow in a completely straightforward logic, and it might not be the most sensitive or thoughtful thing to say."

She had a point. I stopped and thought about it. She definitely had a point.

"You both need to just take a break from this conversation right now," she said, urging me to put a pin in it for the night. "Walk away. Cool off. When he says nonsensical stuff, that's not the fully recovered Dave speaking. You need to give him a break. Give him more time. Look how far he's come, Alli. He's going to keep healing. But you need to just be patient. This? This is not helpful, as frustrating and excruciating as it is. You're right to feel the way you feel. But so is Dave."

Damn it, she was right. She was so right. This was why I had needed her. I was still crying, but I did feel slightly better. "Marya,"

I said, "Rob must think I'm crazy. I'm so sorry for calling you like this."

"First of all, don't be a butthead. And second of all, I am so glad you called. You call me like this anytime, OK? Do you know how much I cried to you when I went through that last breakup? You were there for me at all times. I am here for you now. And I know that things will get better. Just get through today. And then, tomorrow? Just get through tomorrow." I could hear that she, too, was crying by now. She continued: "Right now, that is all that you can do. You can't control anything beyond that. OK?"

"Yeah."

"And call me whenever."

Silence. More tears on my end.

"OK?" she asked.

"OK," I said.

I had to learn to ask for help. To acknowledge that I could not soldier through this one on my own. I had never been ripped open like this, sapped of my strength and stripped of the shiny veneer of confidence and self-sufficiency that I had always been able to present to the world, not as an artificial facade but because, prior to that, I had generally felt like I was in control. That I could handle it—whatever it was.

But in those days, dark as they were in every sense of the word, all I could do was continue to put one foot in front of the other. Those were the days that taught me just how fragile and fickle and entirely out of my control life truly is. My previously held belief that I could work hard and do the right thing and then plan and control the unfolding of my own life? That illusion was yanked quickly and cruelly from my grasping hands, leaving me empty and lost.

Lacy had called this my "ocean time," and now another ocean image came to mind. Growing up, we would take family trips out to the eastern beaches of Long Island every summer. My parents had met out there, bodysurfing during a hurricane in the early 1970s (yes, they had both, independently of each other, slipped onto the beach to swim in the rough surf after it had been closed to the public). Swimming in the ocean was always a huge part of our family trips out to Long Island. We all loved to bob atop the rough Atlantic waves, to try to harness their power to glide weightlessly toward the shore.

But, when you're first getting in, the ocean can be rough, even a bit scary. Especially when you're just a child. There is always that point when you are paddling out that you have to confront the white, roaring wall of breaking water. The Atlantic can be ferocious, and as a kid I was tossed around quite a few times by waves twice my height, spun in the churning swirl of tidal energy until I was inhaling salty water and did not know which way was up.

Still to this day, even after several summers of lifeguarding, I feel that jolt of adrenaline—that mixture of excitement and fear—when I am swimming out through the breaking line of the ocean waves. There's always the risk that a wave will break right on you and pull you into its mayhem. And yet, the only way to make sure you *won't* be smashed by the approaching wave is to swim directly *at* the rough, breaking water. It is counterintuitive and it can feel frightening, but there it is: swim right at the breaking wave, either dive under it or jump over it, but there's no avoiding it. Try to turn back and run away and it will catch you eventually, pulling you down in your futile escape attempt. You have to confront it, you have to go *through* it, in order to get beyond it.

And then, once you are past the breaking line? Bliss. Weightlessness. Peace and quiet, your body bobbing effortlessly atop smooth waters, your view one of tranquil and expansive blue. I had to keep swimming, directly at the breaking line of my fear and my anger and my sadness and my sense of loss. There was no other way to get around this pain other than to keep moving steadily forward. To keep pushing forward and somehow make my way through. And so that's what I did.

A calendar hung right above my nightstand, and each night as I climbed into bed, I would tick another day off, exhaling a sigh of relief. I would think: *I survived; I made it through another day. I am one day closer to . . . to what?*

As tired as I felt, as weary as I would be each night when I fell into bed, my mind would spin for hours. "Three A.M. is your worst enemy," Lee said knowingly, when I complained to her of my sleeplessness.

Each morning I would get up, summoned by the first cries of my hungry baby, feeling heavy, not having slept. I would plod through the darkness to her crib, thinking: *Today is not forever. I just have to make it through another day.*

Dave urged me to remain patient—he told me that we just needed more *time.* He would continue to improve and to heal. I had to remember and acknowledge how far he had come. I had to listen to the insistence of friends and family members who assured me that Dave was still improving; that I was too close to the situation on a daily basis to notice that positive changes were very much still occurring in him. They reminded me of the days when he could not tell me what city he was in, when he could not make it a few hours without the crushing need for a nap.

"Keep writing; writing will save you," Lee told me. She had first said those words to me just days after the stroke, early in the recovery—way too early for me to see or understand the wisdom in them. At that time I had been working on my third novel, *Sisi,* but by then it was mostly just editing that remained. That I could do. That was familiar, a welcome escape, even.

But the creatively taxing work of writing something new? Creating something? I could not fathom it. Writing was where I found my joy. Writing was where I went to play. Writing required space and time and freedom, none of which I had.

And yet. In those exhausting days so many months later, when the fragments of our former life were scattered around us, as trampled and trodden as the late-winter Chicago snow, I returned to these words of advice. *Keep writing; writing will save you.* I returned to the letters that had accumulated on the pages of Dear-Dave.doc. I was adrift—too far removed from the initial event to have any remaining reserves of energy or hope, and yet still too far away from the "full recovery" toward which we had been striving to feel any peace or confidence that we would indeed arrive at that elusive place.

I realized then that I *had* to write. I had to write in order to make sense of what had happened, what was still happening. I have always found that I can best make sense of the world and of intense or incomprehensible situations by writing. It is my way of taking inventory, of sorting, of understanding. That was what I needed right then: I needed to do a major inventory—not just of the days and months right after Dave's stroke, but of the days and months and years that had gotten us to that point. To try to make sense of the present. To try to make peace with the fact that the past felt lost and the future loomed like a vast, frightening unknown.

I would write to understand. I would write to bring together the ragged and disparate threads, to try to weave something comprehensible from the frayed strands of pain and love, loss and hope, fear and faith, beauty and brokenness. I would write to try to find some order, some narrative, some meaning from the daily torment of having lost so much. And so that is what I did. Dear-Dave.doc became the place where I turned, the pages piling up as the days passed, one by one.

Today is not forever, I told myself, time and again. *I am one day closer to* . . . to what? To a time, I hoped, when life would not feel so hopeless.

Our present would change. It, like the Chicago winter, had to pass eventually. I had to believe that sometime, somehow, the sun would break through once more, and the light would return.

Chapter 34

"MOM," I SAID, CLENCHING MY TEETH AS I TRIED TO SWALLOW
the tears. I had to get honest—with myself, with others. It was an
early winter morning, faint light trickling through the windows,
the kitchen smelling like coffee. "I just . . . I just feel complete and
utter despair."

It was a dark thought for me to admit to. Despair, I recalled
from my time as an English major studying Dante, is considered
a major spiritual offense. To despair is to commit a personal
treachery against God; it's a lack of faith, a denial of the gift of
hope, an abandonment of one's belief in grace. And yet here I
was, confessing to my despair.

My mom stared at me a moment, her coffee poised in one
hand. "Alli," she said eventually, her voice forceful in the quiet
kitchen. "This situation is *not* hopeless. What happened to your
faith? You've always had this incredible faith in God. Well, now is
the time to call on that. Lean on God."

Those simple, frank words struck me. My mom had a point.
What use was my faith if not for this precise moment, when I felt

the suffocating grip of despair and doubt? What was faith, really, if not the thing I needed right then, when I had absolutely no proof that things would get better? Wasn't that what faith was— the belief in something unseen, the belief in something whose very existence could be rationally and reasonably denied?

Sure, I could profess my faith and thank God when things were going well—when I had a great husband and a great job and a baby on the way and my health and close friends and a loving family. But that was not *faith* that God was good, really, was it? That was simply a matter of agreeing with the overwhelming and abundant evidence. I needed faith here, when the evidence seemed to point to the fact that life was hard and sad and scary, rather than good and smooth. I needed faith here when the doubt lurked in my mind that maybe God was not here with me, that maybe He had abandoned me—or worse, that He had never been beside me to begin with.

It's like the difference between innocence and purity. Innocence is circumstantial; it is a state of being that stems from a lack of exposure or experience. It's passive rather than active. Purity requires an active choice; it is attained only once the test has come and the test has been passed. Prior to this, I'd had the faith of the innocent. It had been, quite frankly, easy to keep my faith. Why not believe that God is good? Up until that point He had been, well, quite good.

Here, though, was a big old test. Could my faith live up to this test? I thought of the old proverb: *Through hottest fire is forged the strongest steel.* Could I maintain my faith through the heat of this fire; could I make it through the pain of these tests? Could I not only maintain my faith, but allow it to take a deeper foothold in me, to grow stronger—and to make me stronger in the process?

Here was my chance. I was being exposed to plenty of reason

to doubt; I had days when I was angry and sad and confused. I did not understand why this stroke had happened or where we would be going from there, and I certainly did not feel like giving thanks for the trial of it all. I wanted no more of it—I wanted that burden to pass away from me. I wanted things to be good and predictable, like they had once been. I wanted Dave back, like he had once been. I wanted my old life back.

Ultimately, I realized, this was the moment when things between God and me finally got real. This was when I needed to live the faith that I had been thinking, for thirty-one years, that I had been living. I did not understand why the things that had happened had happened. But did I still—even in that place of not knowing or understanding, *especially* in that place of not knowing or understanding—believe that God was with me? Was He there beside me in my pain and brokenness, just as I had always believed Him to be beside me in my joy? Did I believe that God could take this heartbreak and this fear and this fatigue and somehow weave something beautiful from all of the frayed and feeble threads? That there was a divine plan at work here, a much larger picture than the one I could see, a framework that exceeded my capacity to understand?

Yes, I realized. I did. I did still believe that God was beside us. I did, because of so many reasons, so many bright spots that had already shone on us, piercing even some of the darkest places. I had felt God at work, already, in so many moments large and small since that terrible June night on the airplane. I had felt it in the steady hands of Dave's doctors and nurses and therapists, in the peaceful moments while Dave slept in his hospital room, in the faith and friendship of Omar, in the pure and perfect joy of our daughter, in the gentle but immutable strength of my mother-in-law, in the unwavering support of our steadfast community of friends and family, in the ferocious love of my parents and siblings and in-laws and even complete strangers. It was especially in the times of the most unbearable pain that I had seen the most beautiful acts of grace and love, shining forth in sharp relief.

A few years ago, I had a meaningful conversation with Kathie Lee Gifford, a friend and warm supporter of my books and a person whose faith, strength, and generosity of spirit I've long admired. That chat, wonderful for so many reasons, resulted in Kathie Lee sending me a book of daily faith readings—readings that I still close every day with before bedtime. Well, years later, in the dark, wintry days when I worried about Dave's recovery and I worried for our family, I came across a passage in that book from my friend, and it spoke directly to where I was in that moment. I read it multiple times in bed that evening, dog-earing the page so that I could return to it again and again. "The truth is that self-sufficiency is a myth perpetuated by pride and temporary success. Health and wealth can disappear instantly, as can life itself. Rejoice in your insufficiency, knowing that God's power is made perfect in weakness."

The words reached up from the page and hit me in both the mind and the heart. That was it. That was the truth laid out before me. Amen.

A loved one questioned my faith during this time, asking me whether it was scary to rely so heavily on something so intangible, something so impossible to verify. "On the contrary," I answered, "far scarier, in my opinion, is the idea of trying to get through this life *without* relying on faith." Making it through life with only science and proven facts to depend on—that would seem to me like gliding over a ravine without a safety harness. Like trying to get comfortable sleeping on a bed of rocks.

We had met so many angels, hadn't we? There had already been *countless* miracles along the journey of Dave's recovery, and

I could—I would—give thanks for those moments and those angels, while affirming my belief that they would continue to appear for us.

I went deeper in other relationships, too. I went deeper in my relationship with my in-laws and parents and siblings and friends—I ditched the idea of keeping up appearances or acting for the world as if I had it all together, and instead brought an honesty to my relationships that, in the end, strengthened the bonds of those relationships and drew me closer to the people I love. I hugged Dave tighter in the middle of the night. I cherished the new giggles and smiles of our precious baby.

On many nights I went from weeping one moment to looking into my baby's smiling face and laughing. I took photos and videos of Lilly and I shared them with family. "Thank God for her," my mom wrote back. "She's special, Alli. She's a miracle baby. God sent her to bring your joy back." As my father-in-law told me and Dave one morning: "I'm not a spiritual man, but if ever there was something that was going to make me believe in God, it would be that little baby."

It was true; in addition to the brain that was regrowing itself inside Dave's head, we had another little mind that was just opening up and beginning to flower right there in our very home, and she brought with her so many giggles and smiles and feelings of unadulterated joy.

I gave thanks for the unwavering friends and family members who rallied to be by our side and support us. I forced myself to keep the faith that Dave's progress would continue. That we, our little family, would get through it together. That there would be happy days for us on the other end of it all—even if our new idea of "happy" had to also mean "different."

I felt stuck, yes, forced at age thirty to live in a place that felt cruel and foreign. But Dave's brain was not stuck where it was; I reminded myself of that each day, and others reminded me of that on the days when I forgot (and there were many days when I forgot). Dave's brain, like all brains, was plastic, changing, evolving. And the healing, as slow and invisible as it seemed at times, was happening. For his brain. For his body. For our entire family.

Chapter 35

Chicago
January 2015

THE DAY I FOUND OUT I WAS PREGNANT, I RUSHED OUT TO Target and bought a gender-neutral onesie that said "I love my daddy." That evening, when Dave got home from work, I presented him with the gift bag.

"A surprise for you," I said, trying to temper my grin as I gave him the package.

Dave reached into the tissue paper and pulled out the onesie, along with the stick that presented the positive test results—yes, the same stick on which I had peed, but he's a doctor; he's not squeamish about bodily fluids.

"Really?" He looked up at me, incredulous.

"Really." I nodded. "We're going to have a baby."

Dave was thrilled—and completely surprised. He admitted that when he had first seen the baby outfit, for a brief moment, he had assumed out of habit it was a dog outfit for Penny. He had not even thought it possible that I'd know I was pregnant so soon.

The day after my father's presidential announcement, I flew back to Chicago for our twenty-week obstetrician appointment. That morning we had a forty-five-minute transabdominal ultrasound in which we gleaned a thorough view of our healthy baby. We saw everything from the length of the leg bones to the outlines of the ten tiny fingers. It was also during that appointment that our doctor determined the baby's gender, but we opted not to be told that day. Instead, the technician in our doctor's office called a family member with the results. This family member then went and picked up a piñata, filled with candy. When Dave and I gathered with family members that weekend, we hit the piñata and pink candy sprayed all over the room. We could not have been more thrilled to discover that we were having a girl.

Now, a moment of important context here: Dave is the youngest of six boys. Dave likes sports. A lot. Dave had planned to raise a pack of boys, all of them little left-handed athletes whom he would coach in baseball, lacrosse, basketball, football, and anything else they found time to play.

In spite of this conviction of his—or perhaps precisely *because of* this conviction of his—I had come to believe that Dave was destined to have a brood of baby girls. I saw him sitting patiently while one little daughter smeared lipstick across his cheeks and another sprinkled his hair with brightly colored barrettes. I knew my mother-in-law, the mother of all boys, also really wanted to add a baby girl to the ranks of Levys (she confessed after the fact that she'd worn a blue shirt the day of the piñata because she was mentally preparing herself to welcome yet another boy).

"When I first saw that pink candy, I immediately felt this protective instinct," Dave told me. "I've always known very little about women, not having had sisters. It was funny to me to be having a little girl—it was a big growing experience because it dawned on me that I would be having a little girl whom I would introduce to the world. I would teach her, but I would learn about little girls in the process."

That night, Dave read a bedtime story to our two-year-old niece, Annabel. He went over the images on the pages with her, delighting in her pronunciation of the words "banana" and "yellow." I could just see a change in him, and my sister-in-law Erin, Annabel's mom, pulled me aside to tell me what a wonderful dad Dave was going to be.

What I remember from those weeks was just how excited we were. Just how lucky we felt.

Chapter 36

Chicago
June 9, 2015

WE HAD HALF AN HOUR UNTIL WE HAD TO LEAVE FOR THE airport.

I barged into our home office, urging Dave to pull himself away from his laptop and pack his suitcase. "Yeah, yeah, soon, I'm almost done," Dave said, eyes remaining fixed on the computer screen as he shooed me out of the office. He was on a deadline to submit several orthopedic research papers, and he wanted to get them done before leaving for vacation.

Finally, Dave clicked SEND on the last email and pushed himself away from his desk. "I'm going to go for a run really quickly, and then I'll pack," Dave said. He saw my face drop. I am the type who packs the suitcase days in advance, who shows up to the airport three hours before the flight. Dave likes to play what I consider a dangerous game of brinksmanship with the ticket agent, boarding the flight as the plane doors are shutting after a mad dash through the airport.

"Just kidding!" he said, his face breaking open in a teasing smile. "I just wanted to see you freak out. I'll pack now and then we'll go."

How many times since that moment have I wished that Dave went for that run? That he had moved his blood and stimulated his circulatory system and flexed his muscles after sitting still all day. Might he have prevented the formation of that clot? Might we have been able to thwart the stroke that derailed life as we knew it? Would the trajectory of our entire lives have played out in a completely different direction? If Dave had gone for that run—could it have prevented that emergency landing in Fargo? That horrifying night in the emergency room? The harrowing days and weeks and months and . . . might everything have been different?

I'm not sure.

I'll never know.

I'll always wonder.

"If only" . . . the saddest words in the English language.

But Dave did not go for a run that day. For whatever reason, whether it had already happened or would happen in the taxi to the airport or on the plane, the clot formed. We got on that plane as one version of Dave and Alli, and we made an emergency landing, several hours later in Fargo, as an entirely different version of Dave and Alli.

Dave had a stroke when he was young and healthy, when we were expecting our first baby and we were so very happy.

It was a massive stroke, and it nearly killed Dave. He did not die, but our lives changed forever. There is no way to undo any of this, no way to alter that reality.

In the airport security line, Dave had news for me. "I found out that I was selected to be on the resident advisory board for *The American Journal of Orthopedics.*"

I looked at him a moment, pausing a beat, before clapping my hands. "Really?"

He nodded his head, yes. This was particularly satisfying for him because of how much competition there was for this board. Residents did not apply; they were simply selected, which made the appointment feel like that much more of an honor.

This mattered so deeply to Dave because he had spent much of the past three years of residency feeling deeply self-conscious about his abilities as a doctor. No one is harder on Dave Levy than Dave Levy, and he had done a fair amount of self-flagellating throughout residency, and in medical school before that. If he is not perfect, he's convinced he is terrible. If he's not the best, he's convinced he's the worst. With Dave there is no ability to project a veneer of bravado; there's no "Fake it till you make it." It's the best thing about Dave and the worst. It's what makes him work so hard and strive for excellence, but let's just say it isn't always the most pleasant experience for Dave or, say, his wife, when he is going through these self-critiques or crises of confidence.

But here it was, a big, fat stamp of approval. For an affirmation junkie like Dave (I'm one, too; it's probably a large part of why we understand each other so well), it was some deeply satisfying validation from his peers and seniors, the long-withheld gold star that he had been craving for years. The confirmation that all of his hard and honest work was paying off—he was doing a good job.

I looked at him now as we made our way through the security line. "Can we finally put to rest this fallacy that you are a bad doctor?"

He smiled knowingly, nodding after a moment. "Yeah, OK."

After years of self-doubt, Dave was finally beginning to feel satisfaction with all of the work he was putting in. The years of sleepless nights in the hospital, putting himself and his family last after the needs of everyone else, working every weekend and holiday and birthday and anniversary. The years of self-sacrifice and meager pay and school and tests. Dave was finally hitting his stride. Dave was finally getting his groove back. It would all be worth it. We were so close.

We cleared security and found our gate. We ate dinner. We prepared to board our plane, completely unaware that life as we knew it was about to change in the blink of an asymmetrically dilated eye.

When I first told people about this airport security line conversation—one of our last in the final minutes before the stroke—I told it with a sense of the tragedy of it all. Dave was finally feeling good about his career. He was working on a ton of exciting research, and gaining the acknowledgment of his colleagues in doing so. He was finally entering the years of his residency when he would be a senior member of the team; I knew that he would love teaching his juniors, that he would love mastering his surgical skills. And I would love having him around for, say, a few weekends and nights and holidays. We would finally have the time together as a couple that we had longed for. He would be there to delight in our daughter. Dave was finally turning a long-overdue corner; *we* were finally turning a corner as a family.

As Dave's parents said, "You were robbed of the golden period. You were robbed of the joy of your pregnancy, of what should have been your happiest time."

There is a certain amount of tragedy to the timing, it's true. Just as things were about to get really good, they got really bad. I do feel like Dave got robbed of his final years of residency and we got robbed of a joyous period on the cusp of new parenthood.

But now, many months out from the stroke, I can also see it in a different light.

Here we sit in our apartment. It's an unseasonably warm day in late winter. Dave woke up early this morning and worked on an orthopedic paper. Next week, he will fly by himself to a conference in Florida to present on three different research projects. Then he will fly, alone, to New York to meet me and Lilly, where we will spend two weeks on the book launch of my novel *Sisi*. Dave will come with me to launch events and press appointments, and he'll take care of Lilly while I go through the wonderful madness of a book tour. Even just a few months ago I might have laughed dismissively if someone had told me that all of this would be possible.

We went to brunch today with dear friends. Afterward, we walked along Lake Michigan with Lilly and Penny. It was a nice Sunday; it was all pretty ordinary, much like something we would have done in our former life. Except, in one big way, it was different. In the old days, I would not have paused every few minutes to think: *I'm so grateful for this moment; I'm so grateful that we are doing this together.*

When we got home from our walk, Dave was humming a Bee Gees melody and so I pulled up that song on my iPhone and we danced to the recorded version. "Hey, Dave!" I said, clapping to the music. Lilly looked on, amused. "Guess what the name of this song is that you were humming."

"What?" Dave asked, shaking his hips as the music played.

"'Stayin' Alive!' *Ah, ha, ha, ha, stayin' alive! Stayin' alive!*" I pointed at him. "No wonder you have it stuck in your head! You know about staying alive!"

Now, as we sit side by side, our daughter naps in the next room and our dog snores with her head on Dave's lap. Dave remembers our dog once more—boy, does he remember our dog. I'm back to being the third wheel in many of their cuddles, and I could not be happier about it.

I'm reading a book, and Dave is reading from his letters—his "Dave Fan Club" book. He's read these letters before; he read them in July when we first got home from RIC, but he does not remember them. Now, as he makes his way through them again, alternating between laughter and low, emotional groans, it is as if he is seeing these words for the first time. Absorbing the love and admiration that so many people feel for him, steeping in the support that so many loved ones rallied to send his way. It's like he gets a glimpse of his own funeral, a peek at all of the eulogies that loved ones might have written in his honor, only now he gets to weave these words into the fabric of his life moving forward.

As Dave makes his way through the book, I pretend to be interested in my historical novel, but really I'm reading those letters along with Dave. I'm thinking about things, my own mind awhirl. I can hear a bird trilling outside our window—yes, a bird singing, in Chicago, in late winter. That sentence doesn't even make sense as I type it.

A text message comes through on my phone; Margaret asks me how the day is going, how Dave and I are doing. I have answered this same question dozens of times over these past months, but today, for the first time, my answer is different. She asks about the weather, tells me they are having a warm day in Virginia and that she can feel the first hints of spring. I reply: **"It's a bright day here, too, in more ways than just the weather."**

Margaret writes me back that she is grateful to hear it. I am grateful to say it.

When we were in the worst of it, in the days immediately following the stroke, when we did not know whether Dave would survive, Margaret reached out to many friends to ask for their prayers and words of strength. Each one of those letters is a treasure that overwhelms me, makes me weep tears of gratitude and love; I think of one in particular now. It was from a friend of Margaret's—a young woman who, though she does not personally subscribe to a specific faith or religion, took the time to think about this request and send in a beautiful prayer. She wrote:

> *I am seeing a picture. I am seeing Dave opening his eyes and smiling. Smiling because his family surrounds him. I am seeing hands that reach for each other and hold each other, and guide each other to recovery. I am seeing Dave—and his arms hold baby Levy and Alli. They are all together in the sun surrounded by green grass and blue sky and there is love radiating out from them, and around them, and flowing through them.*

I remember so well the first time I read those words. I had been stunned by their simple yet powerful beauty. I had wanted so badly to aspire to that image, the image of Dave being well enough to hold the baby; the image of us, happy, together as a family on the grass in the sunlight. I had loved that image, but in the back of my mind, the louder thought had been: *I wish—oh, how I wish—but I can't really imagine that Dave will ever be well enough to hold his baby, let alone sit outside on green grass in the sunlight.*

If I ever feel the temptation to complain about Dave's progress or recovery, to lament that things are not what they once were, all I need to do is think back to that prayer, to the fact that our outlook was once so grim that I doubted whether Dave would ever be well enough to sit with me and the baby in the fresh air and sunlight. Because, now, he is. He's well enough for that, and for so much more. How far he has come. How far we have come, together.

May we always remember.

I can look at that photo again, the one of us with the four-leaf clovers, without wanting to tear it off the wall and hurl it across the room. The smiles of those two young people, people who have just pledged their lives to each other, young people who imagine a future unfurling before them filled with adventure and love and hard work and joy—those smiles make me smile once again. Sure, maybe now I smile with a film of knowing tears in my eyes, but I can smile.

Spring is returning. After a gray winter, the quality of the sunlight is changing—the bird singing outside our window is a harbinger of more good to come. While once the sky overhead appeared dark and impenetrable, that wall of leaden clouds is now breaking. The air is beginning to feel softer, gentler. One day at a time, I told myself. Day after day, the time passed. Days formed weeks. Weeks formed months. And now winter has to give way to spring. I could not remember how glorious it was—that first sound of a bird on a barren branch outside the window. I forgot. But now I hear it, now I remember.

Book launch is just days away, and I am excited for it. Not only am I not dreading it, I'm actively looking forward to it. I'm remembering book launches from years past and I know that this time around will be different, but I've made my peace with that fact. It will be different, but it will still be good. I've never been more appreciative of the work I love. I've never felt more support and sustaining strength from the community in which I work and the readers for whom I write. I will never forget the way these people rallied to my side. The way they showed up, not as colleagues or customers, but as friends. As compassionate and kind individuals who cared. And the way my loved ones jumped to be by my side so that I could feel supported in this critical moment. I was scared and I was lonely, but I was not alone. Not for a moment.

May we always remember.

I sit beside Dave thinking about the idea of memory, realizing that memory has so much to do with the past, yes, but also with the present. We can and we must remember in the active, present tense of the word. We can remember to always say "I love you" when leaving through the front door, and to say "I love you" when walking back in through that front door.

Our home is lined with photographs—bright spots of joy that we remember from the past. Moments that seem to us, now, to come from a different life. The life before June 9, our life before the stroke. But there will be new moments, too. We will fill new picture frames with new memories—experiences we will imbue with love and joy and meaning. And we will look at them so gratefully, with an appreciation made that much deeper because we know how hard we had to fight in order to live them. We know how close we came to never having those moments at all.

May we always remember to begin the day being grateful for life, however difficult that life may appear. To show up for our loved ones. To listen, to allow them to weep when they need to weep. To cook them dinners when they need us. To be God's angels on this earth just like the angels who showed up for us along our journey through pain.

May we always remember to lavish our precious baby with kisses. To give thanks that she is here and that she is healthy and she is ours—and to give thanks for the fact that we are here to love her and know her.

May we always remember that, even though I spend my days writing about women and their love stories, that ours, the fragile, imperfect, precious story we are writing day in, day out, is the most important one, and that we can choose each day to write it with love and joy and gratitude and faith.

May we always remember, while you treat others and spend your days thinking about the care of the sick, that your life was saved and you are still in this world to help shape it and make it a better place.

Dear Dave, May we always remember how lucky we are.

When you first opened your eyes, you were not yourself. You did not remember all that we had lived through; you did not remember how to speak to me the way you had always spoken to me. You did not remember all that we had wanted for our future. That has come back, with time. What we have between us is once again familiar and worn-in, and yet, in some ways, it is also entirely new and different. It was like you and I had to fall in love all over again. And we did. Our marriage looks different today than it did a year ago, but isn't that the case for any marriage? Isn't marriage a dynamic thing in which two people are constantly growing and learning and evolving—and isn't the key to honor and cherish and nurture your love for your partner even as you grow and learn and evolve? Even through the process of regrowing a brain and fixing a hole in one's heart?

Dear Dave, May we always remember how lucky we are
to have one another.

We are not lucky because life is easy or smooth, or because it makes sense or because we are in control. Life is hard and scary and entirely out of our control, but we know that now. We understand it. We've stared at death—we've confronted the reality that life is fragile and fickle and that no one, not even a world-class neurosurgeon, can tell us what tomorrow brings, or even what the next hour brings.

We've had the opportunity to live out the promise we made to each other on the hilltop right before we found the four-leaf clovers. We've had the chance to live out the vows we made on the day when I pressed the four-leaf clovers and told you that we were lucky.

We are lucky to be living this life.

And best of all is that, for now, we get to live it together.

June 9, 2016

Dear Dave,

You had a stroke one year ago today. A massive, scary, improbable stroke that took us completely by surprise and changed the course of our lives forever.

With your stay in the ICU and your state of amnesia came a series of letters that I decided to write to you, along with the hundreds of letters and emails and prayers that I would collect from so many people who love you.

This is the last letter I am going to write you that will be a part of this DearDave Word document.

After today, we move forward, onto a new, blank page.

I've measured time for a year in relation to June 9, 2015. Everything was bracketed in my mind as either "before June 9" or "after June 9." Every day of this past year I have woken up and looked down at my calendar. First, I would check what it was that we had to do that day. Then, I would scroll back to this day one year prior; I would take a moment of refuge and solace in looking at the simple activities of the same date, before the stroke. I'd recall what we had done, two people in a state of innocence, enjoying the busy excitement of fulfilling work and the early days of a first pregnancy. I'd remember us how we were before that plane ride. Before the fall. Before everything changed.

One year ago today, June 9, was the worst day of our lives.

Today, we are going to celebrate. It's your "Alive Day." Tonight we will take your parents—the first people I called from the ambulance in Fargo—and your family out to dinner, and we will celebrate the fact that you are alive. Your mom called me yesterday, telling me she had bought a balloon for you that said "Welcome back!" We thought that seemed right.

This weekend you and I and Lilly will gather with a group of friends and we will raise a glass to your life and to your loved ones and the community that rallied to our sides one year ago today, and every day of this past year.

When organizing this little get-together, I wrote the following email to our friends, with the subject line "Dave is Alive!":

> Hi friends!
>
> June 9 marks a not-so-fun one-year anniversary for us. We can't think of a better way to commemorate this crappy day than by surrounding ourselves with people we care about.
>
> Please come on over & join us on our rooftop as we raise a glass to our favorite stroke survivor & rehab rockstar—life is good and it's been a remarkable year.
>
> Love,
>
> Alli, Dave & Lilly

It is June in Chicago again. It is the best time of year once more, and the sunshine has returned. I will spend the day reflecting and giving thanks. We have so much for which we can be grateful.

This past week, we published a piece in *The New York Times* discussing a little bit of what we have been through. The piece elicited very strong reactions from the readers, and we've received hundreds of thousands of clicks and countless incredibly thoughtful and moving responses. One email struck me in particular. It came from a young woman who goes to Yale. Her father had a stroke several years ago, and she wrote this to us:

> I'm happy to say that my dad lived through his stroke, and while he is very different from how he was before, he, my siblings, and my mom have only redou-bled our commitment to him and our love for each other. Every day his walking and talking improve, and he smiles very often, especially around our family.

He is very different from how he was before.

We've redoubled our commitment to him and our love for each other.

Every day he improves.

He smiles very often.

That's it, isn't it?

The life we knew, Dave, before the stroke—that's gone. That version of ourselves and our loved ones and that particular path we might have forged is gone. It's all been replaced by something new and different, and perhaps it's a little less innocent and simple. But, as different as the world and the family and the people in it may appear, things can still be good. Life can still be filled with hope and, as this young woman so beautifully put it, with love.

Celebrated neurologist and Holocaust survivor Viktor Frankl said, "Suffering ceases to be suffering at the moment it finds a meaning." I think about that quote a lot. Did we want this to happen? No. Do I feel as though we understand everything that has unfolded and will continue to unfold for us as a result of this stroke? Hardly. Do I feel as though we've been able to draw meaning in all of this? Yes. Every single day, yes. And I know that we will continue to do so.

I hear you in the next room, playing with our daughter as I type these words. Your mother recently confessed to me that, on their midnight plane ride out to Fargo, your father had very seriously prepared her and Andy for the fact that you might die, that it was very likely a flight for all of them to see you one final time and say goodbye. And if you didn't die, we probably could never expect much more for you than a life of complete helplessness and 24-hour care.

I hear you now, in there, playing with Lilly, making her laugh.

I say: thank you, God. Thank you so much for this moment. For the fact that Dave knows Lilly and Lilly knows her father.

That is no small thing.

We never made it to Hawaii. We never had a "babymoon" trip. We got rerouted, and the journey we took instead was one we never expected and one we never would've chosen, but it happened. This year has been lumpy. There have been glorious peaks and ghastly valleys.

Brain injury is so especially difficult on a patient and the loved ones because we can't see the wound in the brain. We can't set it like a broken bone in a cast, we can't watch as a scar slowly heals and diminishes and maybe even disappears. To believe that a brain is healing requires faith; it requires one to submit to time and to patience and to trust—to hope without proof that the unseen is occurring. It requires a deep and abiding faith that, though we can't see it—the mind is doing the miraculous work of regenerating, a million tiny but mighty cells coming alive and coming together, working once more to create miracles large and small, seen and unseen.

All this year, we've heard so much talk about fighting and striving for a full recovery. Everyone hopes and believes you can make a full recovery. I've thought so much about this phrase, these words. I've wondered just what a "full recovery" would mean or look like.

Full recovery. To me, I think there's something in the first word there: "full." I think we need to focus on that. A full recovery, in my opinion, means that you are able to once again live a full life. What does that mean—a "full life"? That's a question that each of us can and should answer differently. But this I know for certain: it does not mean a perfect life. Because that's not possible, and never would have been, stroke or no stroke. Nor does it mean an easy life. A predictable life. We now know that that is not possible, either. A life without long trials and sudden, shocking disruptions does not exist. Not for us, not for anyone.

There are still so many good moments to be had. Life has been beautiful. When I stop to really think about just how beautiful it has been, it becomes a bit overwhelming. I have studied yoga in the rain forest in Costa Rica and I have studied Shakespeare in the Gothic buildings of Yale. I have looked out over the world from atop the Swiss Alps, and I have looked up at the sky while swimming in the Great Barrier Reef. I have fed the homeless in Chicago and have sat down to dinner with two sitting presidents. I have laughed so hard that I was unable to catch my breath, and I have cried so hard that my head felt like it would split apart. I have cradled my newborn baby in my arms and wept; I have cradled my sick husband in my arms and not wept, because I was far too frightened of what would happen if I allowed the tears to begin.

Even, with all of that, without a doubt, the greatest adventure of my life is the one we are living, Dave, each and every day. The greatest story I will ever tell is the one we wake up to and write anew each morning. "Choose to be in your life, to be in your marriage, every single day." That is what the priest told us at my brother Teddy's wedding to Emled, years ago, and though I did not fully understand it at the time, I think that I do now. No marriage is easy. No love is easy. Faith is certainly not easy. Tragedy can come at any time and in any shape. Life gets scary and it gets hard. We scream and we cry and we fall to the floor, railing with fists clenched that we just don't want to do it any longer.

And that is when we have our greatest chances and our greatest choices.

We choose, today, to strive toward a full recovery. A full life must inevitably come with its challenges. But it also means a life full of love and loved ones. A life full of gratitude for both the beauty and the brokenness. A deeper faith and a more meaningful appreciation for every single day that we are given.

Acknowledgment of our blessings and a genuine compassion for those who are struggling. We choose that.

The stroke was sudden and it was painful and it forever changed the road on which we walked. But today, and every day, we must remember to look back and see how far we've come. We see the many steps behind us, and we nod to them with gratitude and understanding. We see the many steps before us, and we look toward them with gratitude and hope. We see that, on our journey, we still stand beside each other, hands intertwined, and we choose to keep moving forward on the new road that stretches ahead.

ONE YEAR AFTER MY STROKE, GRATITUDE IS THE FIRST THING on my mind. I am so grateful to be alive and here with my wife and daughter. It was certainly a scary experience to have almost died, but one positive I can unequivocally point to is that it has truly brought me closer to my entire family. My world has shifted, but the result of that shift is that now I see life from an entirely new perspective. That is such a cliché, of course, but it defines my existence. My entire life is a second turn—a second look, a second attempt at trying to lead a happy and meaningful reality.

It has been more than one year since my stroke, and the only real deficit I have right now—at least that *I* can detect, though my wife might have more to say on the matter when I "forget" to fold my laundry—is in my short-term memory. It is coming back slowly but surely, but it is still an odd experience to feel, in some ways, like a different person. I used to have a memory like a steel trap—almost photographic. I am not saying that I will not get back to that, because I sure hope that I will, but I am having to learn to think through things differently, to make adjustments in life that I never anticipated having to make.

Many, many people suffer strokes. When I was in medical

school, it was, I believe, the third most common cause of death. But not many people suffer strokes at my age. In my rehabilitation group this past year, there was only one person even close to my age, and he had suffered a traumatic accident. That said, strokes in young people are becoming increasingly common, and that's a troubling trend.

I remember learning about the artery of Percheron in medical school and thinking about how unusual it was. We learn about anatomic variants as students, and I have seen plenty, both in medical school and residency. I never imagined myself to be one of the select few who have one of them. But, of course, I do. And nearly all of us have some sort of anatomic variant within us that we do not know about. You probably do, too. It may be one of those random shunts in your heart, one of those odd ducts in your liver, one of those different arteries in your brain. But it is extremely rare that one of those variants would threaten your life. Those variants—the life-threatening kind—were weeded out by evolution, right? We have had years upon years of evolution and have changed in kind—all for the better. But some odd variants come through.

The simple fact is that given the stroke I suffered, there was a good chance that I would not be here right now. That is certainly a scary thought, but, really, it is a reality no different from that facing anybody else; if you suffered a car accident yesterday, you might not be here, either. And therein lies one of the most thought-provoking aspects of my illness—that I have gone through so much yet am really no different from anybody else.

Father's Day in 2015 may have been the most special of all to me. I don't remember a lot of things from my early days after the stroke, but I do remember getting a T-shirt from my wife, who was six months pregnant at the time. It said "Father of the Year" and had a picture of a scene with a father in it from the movie *Finding Nemo*. I still wear that shirt quite often and love showing it off to our little girl. It is an odd experience to be a father after all of this, but, my God, has it been rewarding. I could not have dreamed of a sweeter baby—a more adorable little girl who is so happy and eager to show love. We are about to enter the "stranger-danger" phase of her life, where she might not be as friendly or open with everybody, but it feels pretty good to know that Alli and I will be exempt from that phase.

Perhaps that is the greatest gift that Lilly, and fatherhood, gives us—making us feel so whole and loved and *happy*. That sounds superficial and self-centered, of course, but that is what babies give us—the ability to look at ourselves and to be proud of who we are and the type of father or mother we strive to be. That is essentially the purpose of life—to be the best version of ourselves and to be that way for those we love. And Lilly has helped me find that so easily—and happily. I fall more in love with her every second I spend with her.

In addition to Father's Day, both of our dads celebrate their birthdays in June—the month of my accident. It pains me to think that not only did they have to deal with my mortality, but also they had to do it on their birthdays. Instead of thinking of the many wonderful years behind them, they had to grapple with the possibility of my death. One father had to consider a family with one fewer son, and the other had to consider a daughter made a widow at the age of thirty. But both dads have been so supportive; they are both remarkably loving and strong. They have lived almost their entire adult lives for others, for their children. My dad said last year, "If Dave is here to celebrate with me next year, then that will be all the birthday gift I could want." That's great, because I have not gotten you a gift yet, Dad.

I did not die last year and am now working toward making a full recovery. That is an astounding thought, considering where I was last June. But, if anything, I have really learned of the miraculous power of the human brain. There was one moment a couple of months ago when I could actually feel the healing. I was reading a newspaper but could only identify individual words one at a time. I knew what the words meant, but I could not read complete sentences. It was an exceptionally unique experience, and it was scary. Will this last forever? I wondered. Will I never again be able to read? I worried and worried my way into a nap, and, when I woke up, the words no longer appeared to me like that. I look back on that experience as a healing moment—my brain was changing and adapting to the injury it had suffered. Now I only hope that that experience will happen again and again.

So many doctors, nurses, physician's assistants, and therapists poured their skills, patience, empathy, and energy into first saving my life and then restoring my life, from the Sanford Medical Center in Fargo, across many of the departments at the Rush University Medical Center, and at the Rehabilitation Institute of Chicago. How can I ever fully thank these talented professionals and wonderful people? I cannot; there is no way that they will ever know how deeply I appreciate all that they did for me and my family. But I can try my best to pay it forward with my own work for my own patients, every day.

My friends have been an amazing support network for me through this. I have been visited by people from New York to California, and I could not be happier when I think about the people I have in my life. If the measure of a true friend is one who shows up in your time of need, then Alli and I count ourselves truly fortunate to have many, many true friends. When each one of them visits, I wonder if I am going to somehow make them uneasy or uncomfortable, but they all bring their unique love and encouragement. I still feel like myself; I share inside jokes with each one of them, and it is so great to remember and rehash those jokes. I am a fortunate person, and I cannot dream of a world without my friends.

My family has been through the most difficult of circumstances. They almost lost one of their own at far too early an age. They have had to deal with the recovery of that same individual, who in many ways has been growing up again, from infancy to manhood. But they have handled it so well and have known exactly when to push me and when to love me. We all love our families, but perhaps we do not know how much until one of our family members is in danger. The true colors of family reveal themselves then, and we remember just how remarkable each one of our loved ones is. You understand your family so much more clearly after an incident like this, and I feel such love and gratitude for every single one of my brothers and my parents.

Finally, I want to reflect on the love I have for the greatest gift in my life, Alli. She has been with me at every turn, and I could not have asked for a more incredible companion through it all. She is the absolute best wife anybody could ever hope for. In the "Fan Mail Book" that Alli put together for me, my brother Andy wrote:

At one point, I wrote more—more about my feelings during all this; how hard it was to see you not yourself; how much I love you (I really really love you); how great Alli was—but none of that seems to matter now, except Alli, she really is amazing.

This spring, Alli launched her third novel. While I have loved all of her books, I believe that this one, *Sisi,* is her best work yet, and I was so grateful to be there with her, cheering with Lilly throughout the launch. Lilly and I even got to make a cameo appearance as Alli's groupies when she went on the *Today* show to discuss her work with Kathie Lee Gifford and Hoda Kotb. Alli was so nervous about the launch, how she would juggle everything with a new baby and all of the stress of our current lives, but she made it look easy, as she somehow manages to do with all of life's challenges. In spite of all of her hard work as a writer, Alli always makes her family and her loved ones her first priority. She works every day to bring her best traits to our marriage and to motherhood. Her level of understanding—both of me and of my condition—still staggers me daily, and I simply cannot believe how patient, faithful, affectionate, and devoted she has been through all of this. She has taken over everything in our lives for the past year, and I am ready to start helping her out.

My greatest joy is the little family that Alli and I have started, and the love we have in our home for each other and for our baby girl and, yes, for our "first child," our dog, Penny. I call them "my triumvirate." Alli asked me recently: "If you died today, would you die a happy man?" That might seem like a morbid question, but, after what we have been through, it is not that outlandish a topic for us. My answer was, "Yes, because of my triumvirate." I love them with every ounce of my heart.

I wake up every day amazed that this is the life that God gave me. He somehow brought these incredible women into my life. I am not sure how I would have recovered without my family, but I know that I certainly would not be as strong without them. My favorite nickname for Alli has always been "Angel." If I need to show anybody me at my best, I need to point no further than the angels I have at home.

This June, right around the time of the one-year mark from the day I survived, we took a trip out east to Alli's family's place on Lake Champlain. It is a special place for Alli's whole family, but it is especially meaningful for us because that is the place where I proposed to Alli. This time, we went back with our daughter. On our last night, just before sunset, Alli and I took Lilly up to the hilltop where we became engaged. It was the same time of evening and on a night as clear as it had been, there, before the blue of Lake Champlain and the green of Vermont, when we had first made the decision to join our lives together years earlier. We showed Lilly this place, and we thought about what our promises had meant years earlier and what they still meant as we moved forward, back down from that same mountaintop. You know what we found during that visit to Lake Champlain? Something we had not found since our engagement. Another four-leaf clover. We have decided that that one goes to Lilly. Alli has pressed it and put it on the same photo where we have our other four-leaf clovers, right above the words "May we always remember how lucky we are to have one another."

How does one move on from this? Where do I go from here? Those are the questions I find myself asking every single day. But the exciting thing is that those questions are no different from the questions that anybody else is asking. And, for that, I am and will always be thankful.

—*Dr. David Levy*

About the Author

ALLISON PATAKI is the author of the bestselling historical novels *Sisi, The Traitor's Wife,* and *The Accidental Empress,* as well as the forthcoming children's books *Nelly Takes New York* and *Poppy Takes Paris,* which she co-authored with her friend Marya Myers. She is also the co-author, with her brother Owen, of the historical novel *Where the Light Falls.* Her books have been translated into more than a dozen languages and her work has been featured in news outlets including *The New York Times,* ABCNews.com, *USA Today, Fox News,* and *The Huffington Post.* Pataki and her husband, David, are passionate about raising awareness of the difficulties of life after a stroke or traumatic brain injury. The daughter of former New York State governor George E. Pataki, Allison Pataki graduated cum laude from Yale University with a major in English, and is a member of the Historical Novel Society. She lives in New York with her family. To learn more and connect, please visit:

allisonpataki.com
Facebook.com/AllisonPatakiPage
Twitter: @allisonpataki

About the Type

This book was set in Celeste, a typeface that is designer, Chris Burke (b. 1967), classifies as a modern humanistic typeface. Celeste was influenced by Bodoni and Waldman, but the strokeweight contrast is less pronounced. The serifs tend toward the triangular, and the italics harmonize well with the roman in tone and width. It is a robust and readable text face that is less stark and modular than many of the modern fonts, and has many of the friendlier old-face features.